Acupuncture for
Surviving Adversity

ACUPUNCTURE for SURVIVING ADVERSITY

Acts of Self-Preservation

YVONNE R. FARRELL

Foreword by Russell Brown, L.Ac.

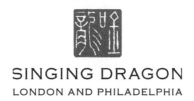

SINGING DRAGON
LONDON AND PHILADELPHIA

First published in Great Britain in 2021 by Singing Dragon,
an imprint of Jessica Kingsley Publishers
An Hachette Company

1

Front cover image source: Nate Bernstein.

A CIP catalogue record for this title is available from the
British Library and the Library of Congress

ISBN 978 1 78775 384 6
eISBN 978 1 78775 385 3

Printed and bound in the United States by Integrated Books International

Jessica Kingsley Publishers' policy is to use papers that are natural,
renewable and recyclable products and made from wood grown in
sustainable forests. The logging and manufacturing processes are expected
to conform to the environmental regulations of the country of origin.

Jessica Kingsley Publishers
Carmelite House
50 Victoria Embankment
London EC4Y 0DZ

www.singingdragon.com

For my niece, Halston. You are an inspiration.

Your struggle for survival and your journey towards healing and self-acceptance have been Herculean and worthy of celebration. Your Hero's Journey has, thus far, been both heart-breaking and awe-inspiring to witness. Never forget you are an emanation of the Light and you are deeply and profoundly loved.

Contents

Foreword by Russell Brown, L.Ac. 9

Acknowledgments 13

Introduction: Gratitude and Survival 15

1. Survival 21

2. Resistance and Self-Preservation 37

3. Five Spirits/Wu Shen 43

4. The Number Nine 61

5. The Sinew Channels 69

6. The Luo-Collateral System 105

7. The Primary Channels 147

8. The Divergent Channels 163

9. The Eight Extraordinary Vessels. 207

Conclusion: Redundancy, Self-Awareness and
the Miracle of Survival 235

References 241

Suggested Reading 243

Index 245

Foreword

I can't fall asleep.

I'm restless. Gripped by a young and unnecessarily rousing anxiety about some patient, or Ghost Point, or any of an assortment of existential crises. I hold out for as long as I can before I inevitably break, and fire off another dramatically urgent-neurotic email to "Doc Farrell," begging for clarity and sedation.

This is how every email I sent to Dr. Yvonne Farrell happened in the eager but terrifying early days of my clinical practice. (Well, a lot of them.)

I had the great fortune of being the eager but terrified student of Dr. Farrell almost twenty years ago. Over these twenty years, Yvonne and I have become colleagues—and friends—and I credit her work with being the foundation of my practice. Her mastery of the complete meridian system—integrating both the Primary and the Secondary Vessels—gave me new eyes. I see the world differently because of her instruction; I see myself differently.

It is only in retrospect that I realize that every question I ever asked in these twenty years—every panicked text in the middle of the night—was always a variation on the same question: *How do you survive adversity?* How do you outpace the seemingly relentless, insurmountable, painful struggles that come with being alive? How do you move forward, and why?

I like to think that when she sat down to write this book, she was writing it just for me, to answer my question, definitively.

This book is primarily about the Secondary Vessels, a subject most acupuncture schools treat like Harry Potter is treated by his Muggle family—crammed into a bedroom under the staircase and told to shhh at fancy dinners. And although there are other books written about them, it is only Dr. Farrell's comprehensive assessment, rendered with practical and personal detail, that definitively pulls them out from under the stairs and declares them neither extraneous nor also-ran.

Dr. Farrell identifies the Secondary Vessels as the essential cornerstone for how we survive trauma; they are critical to how our bodies metabolize, store and move pain so that we may continue to live. But like her last book on the Extraordinary Vessels—which I describe as a memoir hidden within a textbook—this one is also a Trojan Horse: Within its meridian cartography is an unflinching and cathartic meditation on how we rise to meet the inevitability of suffering.

This book is about how our bodies, minds and spirits cope with the crucible of evolutionary stress without becoming lost in pain or going extinct. It is about the grand gift the natural world bestowed on us: a stubborn and awesome predisposition for self-preservation. Which is why I feel it has less in common with a volume of Giovanni Maciocia and more with Charles Darwin's *On the Origin of Species*; or spectacular *National Geographic* reporting on how stars are born, burn for millennia and are then swallowed up whole; or how dinosaurs lived and died.

Yvonne's book is the story of how the things that last, lasted. The beating heart of her writing is survival and the cost of survival: *how living things endure dark days and inclement weather*.

I hope you are brave enough to digest these lessons through the lens of how you survive your own dark days and inclement weather, which we are all doing, even now, even as we hide out reading this book, I hope in some warm corner of Earth. The world itself is holding its breath in survival these days. This is the story of how you survived, too. It doesn't even matter if you never treat another patient again.

I remember receiving her responses on the mornings after those panicked midnight messages. They were usually just a few taut words—tough, loving, wise ones—always a variation on the same, simple reminder: The bad weather is a lesson. The adversary is the curriculum. You will survive this, too. Survival isn't accidental. It's built into your biology. Trust this. Life loves you.

Then she would add, plainly poking fun at my up-all-night neuroses: "What a fabulous opportunity for you!" *That* is Yvonne Farrell. And she was right. She almost always is.

And now we all have this book.

What a fabulous opportunity for us.

Russell Brown, L.Ac.
Summer 2020

Acknowledgments

Writing a book is like becoming a mother. We conceive of something, we gestate it for months or years, first in our minds and then on paper. We labor over it and finally, after writing, re-writing, editing and formatting, we give birth to it. We become a mother.

We are not born mothers; we are nurtured into it. We are created by the experience. Anyone who has ever written knows that the nurturing they receive before they become authors is essential. To that end, I would like to thank those who have nurtured me in ways that were so vital that saying thank you will never be enough. I can only hope that this book will show them how much I love and appreciate everything they have done to help me recover the person I am.

I have had many wonderful teachers in my life but the two who have shaped me the most are Taoist monk Jeffrey Yuen and my dear friend David Chan. They gave me a perspective on Chinese Medicine that has changed me and the course of my life. No amount of thanks will ever be enough and because of you both, I have tried very hard to do the same for others.

To Trace Albrecht, my anchor, my work wife, my dear friend and the person who works so hard to make my life easier, I love you. When life gets challenging, I remember that you and I have managed all kinds of rough times with hard work, internal strength and optimism, some of which comes from tequila or the occasional glass of wine.

Russell Brown, thank you for loving me with honesty. Your willingness to hold me to a higher standard while reminding me that I am already wonderful is a priceless gift. Thank you so much for writing the foreword for this book. Your writing is inspiring and always reminds me to be braver.

They say if you want to learn something in a deep and life-changing kind of way, you should teach. Thank you to my students for your willingness to receive, your curiosity, your frustration and your resistance. I am especially grateful to my Mentorship students. This book is possible because your thirst for understanding gave my broad vision some much-needed focus. A special thank you to Kyla Drever for your writing and editing skills. I have learned much from your advice and support.

Last in the acknowledgments but first in my heart, thank you, Nate. Your brilliant mind and enduring love have done more to make me who I am than anything or anyone else in my life. Mothering you is a privilege for which I am eternally grateful. You are a miracle and I could not be prouder of the man you are.

INTRODUCTION

Gratitude and Survival

We are more than the sum of our body parts. We are the sum of those parts plus every experience we have. We are living, breathing, dynamic systems that express themselves physically, emotionally, mentally and spiritually. We are the recipients of the bounty and the baggage of previous generations. We live in the shadow or light of the families and cultures in which we are raised and we are all connected.

We have the capacity to survive through countless acts of self-preservation. Beyond survival, we are blessed to have in us the ability to learn and grow from most every challenge we encounter in life. When we have alignment in our constitution and temperament, and our resources are plenty, we are ensured the building blocks needed for us to thrive in a life of meaning and purpose. We are able, with attention and intention, to become more of who we are. We can illuminate and embrace the lost or hidden parts of ourselves so that we might become a more authentic expression of that Self. Every movement we make towards consciousness makes us more human, and it is the depth of that humanity that will support us in fulfilling our purpose in this life.

As Carl Jung said, "The reason why consciousness exists, and why there is an urge to widen and deepen it, is very simple: without consciousness things go less well" (1975, para. 695).

I am a big fan of Pema Chödrön. I especially like her teaching around the quality of Maitrī. Maitrī means benevolence, loving-kindness, friendliness, amity, goodwill and active interest in others. It is the first of the four sublime states and one of the ten pāramīs of the Theravāda school of Buddhism. Maitrī is the practice of developing an unconditional friendship with yourself. It is the gift of self-acceptance. To move beyond survival into a state of thriving, it may be essential to develop a more friendly and compassionate relationship with yourself. I am not talking about cutting yourself slack when you don't feel like doing what needs to be done. I am also not talking about having lower expectations of yourself. I am advocating for us all to be as kind to ourselves as we are to someone else who is clearly suffering. When you are struggling with life, do you have compassion for yourself or do you hear all of those critical voices from the past, judging you harshly for your choices and actions?

With practice and intent, we can accept our current struggles and recognize that the choices and actions we have made to get to this point were, by and large, unconscious acts of self-preservation. We do what we must to get through life's challenges and stresses, but mostly we do that without thinking it through or even realizing the potential cost of the decisions we make. When we do think it through beforehand, those thoughts are typically formed by unconscious biases and habituated or indoctrinated beliefs. If we were told often enough that we are unworthy, we will believe we deserve what is happening to us, and our thoughts and behavior will align with those beliefs. We typically do whatever we believe will get us through what we are facing in the moment.

It is a valuable endeavor to practice gratitude for this gift of survival. If we are currently alive, then our active impulse did everything it could to keep us that way. If this impulse can manage to keep us alive long enough, we may, in time, be able to see that we deserve better. If we are still alive, we may be able to see that we can have more, that we deserve more, that we can be more or, even more poignantly, that we are enough. That is truly something to be grateful for.

When I look into images of Pema's face, I see that kindness and self-acceptance, and I am inspired to be more. I can accept that the struggle, pain, fear and resistance in my life were part of being where I am now. I can be grateful that I have a survival instinct. I am aware in moments of ease and grace that judging myself as weak, undisciplined or "less than" is an unconscious habit and those voices do not really help me become that person I want to be. I have never seen self-judgment make anything better. I know that it is possible to be kind to myself and still challenge myself to strive for being more of who I am.

I have watched my patients find many ways to survive. I have seen them somatize, repress, suppress, deny and resist suffering in every and any way possible in order to get through the tragedies and challenges that are derailing them from the lives they want to have. I am always saddened by how harshly patients judge themselves for the results of those acts. It is heart-wrenching to watch someone have expectations for themselves that are so much higher than they would have for others. It is difficult to see the brokenness of perceived failure in their eyes because they are unable to recognize and appreciate the gift of time that they have given themselves because of those actions. When you look into the eyes of someone in that place of self-judgment and you say to them: "You did everything you could to get to this point. You are alive and that means you are already successful. Your body and mind took experiences that were so hurtful, overwhelming and inherently damaging and they dealt with them in the best way they could. Now let's see if we can figure out how you can have more"—when you affirm that, what you see is hope.

This book was written to provide a framework for understanding how effective the channel system is at supporting survival. Within this system, we have layers and layers of function that may be very specifically directed for survival purposes. From the Sinew channels that brace for impact, to the Dai mai which acts as a repository for unprocessed trauma, we have many ways to survive life's challenges and traumas. We have a system that works so hard to keep us alive that if it cannot rid us of a toxic or life-threatening experience, it will find a way to store that experience someplace in the body that reduces our interaction with that challenge. This is an act of creating latency or hiding a problem, so we don't have to deal with it directly or immediately. Each channel system has a way of doing that so that we have time to gather our resources and figure things out. In this book, we will look at why latency is created, how it is created by the different channel systems and what is the cost of creating that latency. If the gift is survival, what is the cost of that gift? We will explore how the Sinew channels, Luo-collaterals, Primary channels, Divergent meridians and finally the Eight Extraordinary Vessels function to keep us alive and what they do to create latency when their healthy function is overwhelmed.

The book has nine chapters and that is no accident. The Heart channel has nine points and its protector, the Pericardium, also has nine points. The Heart's capacity for compassion and unconditional love and the vulnerability that is required from the Pericardium to share that love is at the root of every word I have written. This is a love letter to my students, my patients, my friends and my family. Your ability to survive amazes and intrigues me and I am deeply and profoundly in love with your humanity.

My hope is that it is possible for us to determine where the latency is created, release it and help our patients reclaim their resources. The less we hide from ourselves, the more access we have to who we are and why we are here.

We will be talking about trauma, but this is not a book about trauma. This is a book about our ability to actively survive trauma through acts of self-preservation. I hope the reader will see that this book is about having gratitude for the miracles that are possible when we survive long enough to be able to accept who we are. I hope we will be able to recognize that our humanity is not injured by the events of our lives. We do not need to find ourselves. We need to remember who we are. Releasing the latency caused by self-preservation is like lifting the veil that obstructs our ability to see the truth of our humanity. When we engage in acts of self-preservation, we distance ourselves from our truth. That act may be necessary for survival but it need not be permanent. We can regain our sovereignty. We can let go of victimization and self-loathing and we can take the time gifted to us through those acts of self-preservation to rally the troops and regain the throne. Thank you for reading the book, but before you go any further...grab your crown.

---- CHAPTER 1 ----

SURVIVAL

Humans are remarkably engineered for survival. We are equipped with many biological responses that work to ensure that we can survive even the most challenging or threatening experiences. We are even neurologically hard-wired to avoid behavior that might possibly lead to survival challenges. Yes, human beings have neurological programming that resists change. We are, by nature and often by necessity, risk-averse, often to the point that any change that involves the unknown may be perceived as threatening.

Change, no matter how necessary or logical, is often perceived by the instinctual part of the brain as a potential threat to our capacity to survive. Now, at first glance, we may think that this is a useful and necessary quality to have, and it is. It's like having a Mission Impossible Command Computer in our brain whose prime directive is to keep us alive by telling us where to go and what to do to avoid danger. "Stop!" "Stay!" "Run!" "Fight!" "Look smaller!" "Look bigger!" "Look aggressive!" "Look harmless!" These commands are sent out before we even have a chance to think about what is happening, because if we take the time to think, we may not respond fast enough to avoid the threat. It's a beautiful expression of efficiency in a dynamic system.

It is important, however, to be able to examine what happens when this useful function goes awry. We must acknowledge and even anticipate the potential for failure. There are many ways this system can fail and some of them are complex. People who study the brain are still struggling to fully understand how this and other neurological systems work. How, then, do we, who are not neurologists, have a chance of understanding this system so we might have it work in our favor? We need to find a way to envision this system so that we can see when it is functioning well or when it is failing to do the job. We also need to be able to recognize that not all threat is real. It would also be helpful to be aware of the price we pay for this function.

How do we define survival? Let us, for the sake of conversation, define survival as the continuation of life or existence. Survival is about maintaining enough function to keep you alive. Survival is not about quality of life. It is not about finding meaning and purpose. It is not about expressing yourself in a creative or spiritual manner. It's about keeping your heart beating. It's about your lungs bringing enough air into your body to sustain life. It's about providing enough blood flow to the brain to maintain a minimal level of consciousness. It is about the ability to direct your resources for the specific functions that will be needed to keep you alive in the moment.

Is that enough? I am certain that at some point in my life I would have answered, "Yes, that is enough." There have been times in my life when maintaining minimal function was all I could manage and staying alive was a priority. But now that I am older and facing less life ahead of me than what has come before, I would qualify that answer. I would now say, "It is temporarily enough." Survival mode is an emergency setting. When we stay in survival mode long-term, there are diminishing returns. We begin to see a decrease in quality of life and an increase in the potential for chronic, degenerative diseases. The important relationships in our lives are affected by this minimal existence. It is very challenging to sustain any level of intimacy in a relationship when your brain is seeing danger everywhere. Many people who have struggled through periods of their lives while stuck in survival mode know that there are worse things than dying. They know you can feel dead and still be alive. This is not how we are meant to live.

We are meant to face danger with a level of hyper-alertness and response, and then, when the danger recedes, we are meant to go back to our relaxed settings. What are the factors that impede our ability to act appropriately in the face of threat and then reset to normal after the threat is alleviated? This question is well worth investigating because it implies that there is a possibility that this survival response is not always working in our favor. If we are constantly living in a state of anticipated threat, if we are seeing danger everywhere, then we are wasting resources that are meant for actual emergencies. We are stuck in a state of defense.

Allostasis is the ability of the body to respond to stress and then, when the stress is over, restore homeostasis. We now know that people can build what is called *allostatic load*, which is evidence that the body is unable to reset to normal after stress. When this system fails to reset to its relaxed setting, allostatic load builds and the long-term result is suboptimal function that, sadly, becomes a new normal. This is how chronic disease occurs. It may also be one of the ways that hormones become dysregulated. It can cause the immune system to become weakened or overactive. Basically, failure of this system to reset has a deleterious effect on the quality of life.

A failure to reset to the relaxed setting may be caused by frequent activation of the high-alert stress response. If we are exposed to stress or trauma over and over again, eventually the system will get stuck. For example, if a child is being bullied at school every day, they are activating this system to survive both physical and emotional threats to their existence. Eventually, the system will get stuck, and even when they are safely at home after school, they will be on high alert, making it impossible to relax. They may have trouble eating or sleeping. Or they may find themselves acting out against their parents or siblings based on some perceived threat. Over time, this can lead to even more serious physical and emotional illness.

We might see the development of eating disorders, or depression and anxiety that lead to self-harm or the need to harm others. Sadly, it is common to hear in the news of young people killing themselves or going on shooting rampages after extensive bullying. These young people are suffering so intensely that survival is no longer a viable priority.

Some threats to survival are so immediately overwhelming that the system remains in survival mode much longer than is necessary. If one experiences major life-threatening trauma or even witnesses it, the ability to reset after the trauma may be delayed. This delay may be a result of the complicated emotions that must be processed following these experiences, such as grief, rage or survivor's guilt. It may also be a result of the dissociation that occurs from shock. When patients experience shock, the circulation is affected. Qi and blood scatters. This scattering of resources and directed qi movement make it difficult to process experience. To survive these overwhelming experiences, we might "check out" for a period of time. During this time, we do not have access to the ability to process the experience so that we can learn, grow and move on.

Nutrition, lifestyle and emotional predispositions can impact how this system responds. When we do not eat well or live well, we create an internal environment that triggers the stress response. When our lifestyle is out of balance, we are more vulnerable. If we do not get enough sleep or if we do not take a vacation when we need it, then we risk the activation of this stress response. These days, I think we must actively seek environments in which we can relax. We might spend time in nature, we might meditate, we might go to the spa or maybe we find our relaxation in the company of others. We might find the reset by sharing a meal with people whose company we enjoy. We might find it in gathering with like-minded souls and engaging in any activity that reminds us that life is worth living.

In terms of emotional predisposition, we know, for instance, that Chinese Medical Theory acknowledges that there are personality types that are, by nature, more vulnerable to stress. For example, Gall Bladder deficiency types are, by nature, timid and more easily startled. They are going to perceive threat more quickly and they will find it much more difficult to reset after trauma. Someone who has a more robust constitution, such as a Type A personality or an adrenaline junkie, is going to perceive threat or stress in a completely different way from the Gall Bladder deficiency constitution. Some people are better built for stress. Although that might seem like a good thing, those hardier constitutions are often capable of ignoring actual threat or changes in their nervous system until the damage is so great it is impossible to ignore. This is why someone who is seemingly healthy and actively engaged in life might suddenly die from a heart attack without even realizing their heart is not functioning optimally. There are so many factors that impact how any individual will respond to the perception of threat.

Birth trauma and intergenerational trauma can also impact how this system functions. These things may predispose us to respond to stress in a less than helpful manner. If you come into the world in a traumatic way, let's say prematurely or perhaps with the umbilical cord wrapped around your neck, then you may have a very early activation of this system that is beyond what might occur in a relatively normal birth. Every one of us experiences some trauma during birth. Coming into the world is a shocking experience, but that shock can be overcome by love and bonding with our mothers or primary caregivers. This may not be so easy if the birth trauma is more severe or if the trauma requires us to be removed from the care of our moms. Intergenerational trauma may also have a very powerful impact on how we perceive the world around us. For instance, there are certain types of mood disorders that "run in families." We might see a patient who is suffering from anxiety with no apparent cause. Their life is going well, they are safe and cared for, their lifestyle is healthy, and they have not, to their knowledge, experienced trauma. How, then, do they come to this state? These patients will usually be able to tell you that their parent, grandparent or even great-grandparent suffered from the same condition. Their brains are being influenced by the unprocessed trauma of previous generations. What is not resolved may be passed down to future generations as a genetic shadow. This is information or experience that is genetically transmitted. The person on the receiving end of this transmission must recognize the influence of that trauma before mitigating the impact it has on their nervous system. If you are the great-grandchild of a slave or Holocaust survivor, part of your brain carries the genetic information of those family experiences. In addition to carrying that information in your genes, it may be that you heard stories in childhood that further imprint that trauma onto your psyche. If you are aware that you have this imprint and that it is affecting how you respond to stressful situations, then you have more choice in how you deal with that.

The potential for getting stuck in survival mode is the major downside of this system. Failure of this system may mean living from the perspective that life is scary and minimal function is acceptable. Nobody consciously chooses this. People who are stuck in this mode are doing the very best they can with a threat they perceive to be real. No one knowingly chooses to develop an auto-immune disease or some chronic degenerative condition after trauma. Nobody wants to be anxious, worried or depressed. Anyone suffering from post-traumatic stress disorder (PTSD) cannot possibly want to accept that this is how their life is meant to be. People end up this way because their brain is trying to keep them alive. That survival response is desperately trying to preserve enough function to keep going. They have come to this place through acts of self-preservation. These acts of self-preservation are largely instinctual or habitual. The way out of this survival mode is bringing consciousness to the process and unblocking the habitual patterning that impedes growth. We need to better understand what we are doing and why we are doing it.

I had thought at one point in the writing of this chapter that I would jump on the *"fill-in-the-blank* for Dummies" bandwagon.

"Survival for Dummies" is, after all, a catchy chapter heading. But the more I thought about it, the more I realized that when it comes to survival, if we are alive, then we are not dummies; we are masters. The problem is not survival; it is the lack of thriving. Even though we are masters at surviving, it is mostly done unconsciously, habitually or reflexively. This means we have little choice to move beyond survival into a state where we are thriving until we can become more conscious of how or why we have survived so far. Surviving gives us the time and opportunity we need to find meaning and purpose, but the skill sets of survival are not the same ones we need to thrive. Staying alive is essential if we are ever to have a chance to explore the deeper questions of our existence, but the ability to survive cannot answer those questions. In fact, getting stuck in the survival instinct is in many ways the opposite of the desire or drive for meaning and purpose. The instinct to run, hide or fight for survival is engaged before the intellect can ponder what the threat is or if the threat is even real. When one feels threatened, whether the threat is actual or perceived, one does not have the luxury of time to ask existential questions like "Why am I here?" "What is my purpose for being?" "Does God exist?" and my personal favorite, "Is this it?" These questions require time and the desire to examine the deeper recesses of being-ness. One does not ponder if one is capable of compassion or unconditional love when bullets are flying overhead; one ducks.

"In nature, when a laboring animal feels threatened or disturbed, the stress hormone catecholamine shuts down labor" (Lothian 2004, p.4). The same is true in laboring women. If a laboring woman does not feel safe, catecholamine levels increase, and labor slows or stalls until she feels safe. This all happens automatically. Laboring women do not think to themselves, "I am feeling unsafe, I think I will slow this whole process down, so it takes longer." Almost anyone who has ever labored in childbirth will tell you that all we are thinking about is getting this whole thing over with, not slowing it down until we feel safe. Emotionally, we want the whole thing done and over with, but, reflexively, the nervous system is saying, not now, it is too dangerous. When a woman feels unsafe in labor, it is almost impossible to engage the intellect and calm down enough to assess the situation rationally. The survival instinct is in charge. That is why it is so important to have a birth plan that has considered what will be needed to help the mother-to-be feel safe. In 1990, I had my son at home. My family thought I was nuts. They could not understand why I would do something that they considered needlessly risky and maybe even irresponsible. I, on the other hand, knew myself well enough to know I would not feel safe in a hospital. I knew I would never feel safe with anyone telling me what to do and when to do it. I was very fortunate to have magnificent midwives who only stepped in when I asked for help. These women helped me feel safer by empowering me to ask for what I needed, and they gave me all the information I needed to make my own choices. It was the right choice for me, but many women will feel safer in a hospital and that is where they should have their babies. The feeling of safety is what matters. When we feel safe, it is easier to find meaning and purpose in the experiences we are having. Having my son was the most empowering experience of my life and I am pretty sure that was at least in part because I felt safe at home. The feeling of safety I found at home allowed me to let go of the fear and recognize the miracle of giving birth. I am aware of how lucky I was to have an uncomplicated and unmedicated birth—not every woman has that experience—but I am convinced that, for me, it was possible because of the sense of safety.

THE TRIUNE BRAIN

What follows is an extremely simplified version of the theory of the three major parts of the brain. This theory was an accepted model of the evolution of the human brain and behavior, proposed by Paul D. MacLean in the 1960s. Although some of what he proposed is now disputed, the functions of the three basic areas of the brain are still widely accepted. He divided the brain into the reptilian, mammalian and human brains based on evolution. When it comes to managing life, it is basically a dance or negotiation between the functions of these three areas.

The reptilian brain, which is said to be the oldest in terms of evolution, includes the brain stem and cerebellum. This part of the brain controls the vital functions associated with survival, including heart rate, respiration, body temperature and balance. The reptilian brain is reliable, but it is narrowly and rigidly focused on survival. It is known as the part of the brain that governs the four Fs: fight, flight, feed and fornicate. We can easily make a correlation between this part of the brain and the function of Wei qi.

The next stage of evolution is the mammalian brain. The limbic system, hippocampus, amygdala and hypothalamus are part of this area. This section of the brain controls our memory of behaviors, emotions and value judgments. If, as a child, you touch something hot and burn yourself, your mammalian brain stores the experience, along with the judgment and emotions associated with the pain. In other words, "that was a really painful experience and I do not want to do that again" is stored in your mammalian brain. This is related to the function of Ying qi.

The most recent stage of neurological evolution is called the human brain or neo-cortex. The neo-cortex is responsible for higher thinking or executive function. It is how human beings developed language, the capacity for abstract thought, imagination and consciousness. It is the basis for human culture, and it is incredibly flexible in its capacity for learning. This is the function of Yuan qi and the connection between Shen and Zhi.

These three parts of the brain are not separate. They are connected to each other through neural pathways that allow one portion of the brain to influence the others. The emotions of the mammalian brain can influence the reptile brain's need to control survival. Accessing the neo-cortex of the human brain with intention can influence the emotions and value judgments that reside in the mammalian brain. How, then, can we create a balance in the dance between the part of the brain that is focused on the four Fs and the part of the brain that is capable of higher thinking, language and imagination? Especially, when the area between those two is responsible for the memory of experience imbued with emotion and value judgments. It is a complex dance and one might ask, "Whose turn is it to lead?"

WEI, YING AND YUAN QI

Each of the three brains has a resonance with one of the three levels of qi. The reptilian brain and its survival function are equated with the defensive nature of Wei qi. The mammalian brain corresponds to the interactive nature of Ying qi. The higher function of the neo-cortex is related to Yuan qi. As we explore the self-preservation capacity of the channel systems, we will see how the function of the triune brain is elegantly replicated in the ability of the channel system to create latency for survival at the three levels of qi.

If we look at the channel system from the perspective of levels of qi, we can see that it offers us numerous opportunities to protect ourselves from threat. It can serve to protect us from external threat through the function of Wei qi. It is designed also to respond to internal imbalances that impact our ability to digest life, interact with others and provide the nourishment for life through the function of Ying qi. It also provides us with opportunities to protect, preserve and acknowledge our identity and belief system, through the function of Yuan qi.

Wei qi (defensive qi) works to defend us from whatever is outside and may be attempting to get in. We typically think of this in terms of the exogenous pathogenic factors. Wei qi protects us from the weather (wind, cold, heat, damp, dryness and summer-heat). In that sense, we are thinking of Wei qi as a sort of external expression of our immune system. True as that may be, it is also a very narrow view of the functions of this remarkable expression of qi. As the most exterior expression of qi, it is both a filter and a mediator between our internal terrain and the world outside. It filters every external piece of information that is trying to make its way in through the skin, through the sense organs and through the Fu (yang) organs. Wei qi filters and determines the level of threat for everything we see, smell, hear, taste, touch and swallow. So, yes, that means exterior pathogens, but it also means everything we eat and drink, everything we experience through our senses and everything that touches our skin...everything. What have you consumed today? What have you touched today or what has touched you? What have you experienced through your senses? What have you reflexively rejected because it is deemed a threat? Whatever it is, your Wei qi responded to it.

Ying qi (nutritive qi) protects us from the painful or emotional interactions that most often occur in relationships. At this level of qi, we are usually trying to protect ourselves from the judgment and expectations of others, but also from the pain of failure and the suffering associated with loss. This is the level of qi where we see emotions having their most obvious impact. Emotions here are specific; we are aware of them and they are beginning to make us uncomfortable enough to want to suppress them. Ying qi nourishes our ability to engage others. Anyone who has ever been in a relationship knows the emotional experience of Ying qi.

When we reach into the inner sanctum of our beingness, we are accessing Yuan qi (source qi). At this level of qi, we are typically trying to preserve our sense of Self. We are trying to hold on to our identity in the face of trauma or challenges to survival. Here we see the embodiment of beliefs. In pathological states, these beliefs are often lies, or at the very least mistaken or unhelpful. These beliefs can serve to keep us alive but not necessarily thriving. This is the level where we see the constitutional component of our immune system. What innate strengths or weaknesses have you been given to support or direct your survival? This level of qi is the catalytic force needed to spark action. If our beliefs are healthy and in alignment with who we are, then the Yuan qi will initiate right-action and support healthy function.

When we are overwhelmed by experiences, each of these levels of qi has an associated channel system that may be engaged to remove the threat. If the threat to survival cannot be removed, then these systems will divert and hold that threat away from the vital functioning centers that keep us alive. These systems have specific aspects that are designed to create and then maintain this latency for self-preservation. When a system creates latency, it is doing one of the things it is designed to do, but it is not meant to do this long-term. The problem with creating latency is that, once created, it must be maintained until the threat can be removed. That means that vital resources that might be used for other things, such as growth and development, are now being used to keep the threat at bay. If we understand the functions of these systems and we can recognize where latency has been created, then we can use these systems to release that latency so that patients can come back into balance. We have at our disposal an understanding of defense and survival which reflects in the body what is happening in the brain. We do not need to fully understand the neurology of it all because the neurological function or dysfunction manifests in physical and psycho-emotional patterns. This is the body-mind.

It is a gift that our medicine gives us. This is an approach that says survival is good but not enough. Once restored, this deep connection in the body-mind can bring meaning and purpose back into our lives.

THE COST OF SURVIVAL

There are people everywhere in the world who live in circumstances that are constantly threatening. Perhaps they live in an area of conflict where violence and death are everyday experiences. Maybe they live with an unpredictable alcoholic spouse or parent. Maybe they live in a society that sees them as something less than human, not deserving of life or liberty. It is likely that, for these people, survival is a priority, so there is often not enough time or resources for pondering meaning.

For those of us fortunate enough to be living in a place where potentially life-ending threat is minimal or infrequent, we may still be stuck in survival because the threat doesn't need to be real. We only need to believe that our environment is unsafe to trigger the need for survival. If we watch the news every day, we are probably going to feel some level of threat. If we live in a place that has significant sensory input, our brains may have become overstimulated and hypervigilant. If that system is frequently activated, there is an increased likelihood that we will be stuck in that state and that fear response will become habituated. This can set us up for the new normal that threat is everywhere. We become stuck in the survival response and we are unable to reset. Now we have a less than optimal "normal" setting. This is one of the downsides of this survival response. Once we are stuck in it, we fail to recognize it and we think that our stress, hypervigilance, paranoia, intensity are what is needed to face each day and survive it.

Years ago, when my father was dying, I learned one cost of survival in a way I never expected. He was in the hospital with metastatic cancer and he had just had surgery to have a rod placed in his spine to try to preserve his spinal cord function. His cancer had invaded his spine and caused several vertebrae to collapse, compressing his spine. He was in agony. There are no words to describe how hard it was to watch him suffer this excruciating pain. I will never forget the day one of his nurses pulled me aside and said, "I don't know how much longer your dad has. No one can predict that. What I do know is that he is in terrible pain and he will continue that way until he dies or you remove him from this hospital. If you engage hospice care, they can better manage his pain and that may give you more time with him." I asked how it was possible that doctors in a state-of-the-art hospital were unable to manage his pain, and she said to me, "Our job is to keep him alive." They would not, could not, risk his life by possibly giving him too much pain medication. The cost of his survival was unimaginable pain and suffering. Not just for him, although that was more than enough, but for all of us. Once we left the hospital, we had ten more weeks with my dad. I spent a lot of that time with him wondering about quality of life and I suppose that is a subject that is foremost in our minds when we or someone we love is dying. But isn't quality of life something we should be thinking of and aiming for long before the dying is inevitable? Can we not find an equitable balance between survival and thriving?

Another cost of survival is the loss of access to our resources. Once we have diverted our resources for survival purposes, we can no longer direct them towards thriving. Creating latency not only keeps pathogens away from the organs but it also requires us to dedicate those resources for the maintenance of that latency. The longer we maintain the latency, the more resources are used, and the more likely we will develop some chronic, degenerative condition that makes life challenging. So...not thriving.

We balance the need for survival with as much quality of life as we can muster. Quality of life can be difficult to define and it changes with age and circumstance, but we know it when we have it.

Cancer, for instance, is a huge life-changing or life-ending challenge, but every day we face other threats to our survival that are real or perceived. How, then, do we survive those threats and what quality of life can we achieve and maintain in the face of those threats?

The channel system of acupuncture is an exquisite representation of the dance. It is an incredibly complete and beautifully elegant way to see and treat the impact of the experiences and choices we make, consciously or unconsciously. Within the system and its diagnostic parameters, we can see how entrenched our life's experiences have become. We can see the price we are paying for our acts of self-preservation.

We have dedicated our lives to a system of medicine that gives us the tools to recognize the problem and provide the much-needed wisdom through treatment and lifestyle counseling that may help patients become more conscious of their choices and regain their sovereignty. We can help patients reset that threshold of response and move from survival into thriving. Like a well-trained dance instructor, we can help patients to manage the dance between survival and thriving.

CHAPTER 2

RESISTANCE AND SELF-PRESERVATION

C hange is inevitable but change is hard and also unpredictable. Change, therefore, may be perceived by the Wei qi as dangerous. This is actually a useful reptile brain function. The resistance to change forces us to stop for a moment, take a breath, engage the Ying qi and the Yi/thought. We are then able to put our attention on the specific threat. We can think about the nature of that threat and we can do a risk assessment. The process allows us to take the time to decide what we are willing to risk in order to change.

Of course, when one's life is in danger, there is no time for that mental exercise. If we are being chased by a fire-breathing dragon, we do not stop and take a breath. We do not engage Ying qi and think about whether or not the threat is real. We push all the energy we have into the sinews and we run. If we have faced our own version of the dragon and we have survived it, we have now trained the Wei qi to respond to the world in a way that recognizes not only the existence of dragons but also the likelihood of being eaten by one. We see dragons everywhere or we anticipate their arrival at any moment. Now imagine that the dragon is sexual abuse in childhood or two military tours in Afghanistan. Those dragons will follow us wherever we go.

Maybe we weren't chased by the dragon. Perhaps in our childhood, we heard the dragon whispering in our ear, over and over again, "You are a waste of space." "You are living on borrowed time." "You are an abomination." That dragon's voice is then carried into adulthood and heard between the lines of every conversation we have. That dragon and its whispering voice are ever-present. The dragon is waiting for us, no matter where we may go. We cannot run from it because it is inside of us.

How, then, do we deal with the dragon? Our instinct is to find a way to make life more predictable. Predictability means safety. Unfortunately, that means we need to become more habituated in our behavior. We need to be able to count on what we already know. We need to rely on what has worked in the past. We need to reduce risk. We need to be able to figure out how to avoid waking the dragon. Change does not have a place in that process and so we resist it.

Even when we are aware of the need for change, which is by no means assured, we are still going to be dealing with the fear of the unknown and the entrenchment of the old habits. If we cannot be sure that change will make things better, then why change? If what we are doing has worked, even if it is not optimal, why risk the possibility of the pain and suffering that is often part of the change process. There are so many things to overcome in the face of that resistance, including a lack of faith in our ability to change, exhaustion, a lack of resources, or we might not even see the true benefit of change. So we resist and typically we do that without putting too much thought into it. It's as if we have an auto-setting that says "No" to change before we can even ponder why change might actually be a good thing. We do this so we can survive.

The cost of survival is varied but it frequently manifests as slowly developing chronic disease. Once we are aware that there are dragons in the world, we adapt. We start to create patterns of behavior or response that are predicated on the knowledge of the dragon's existence. This adaptation often comes in the form of latency creation. We have experienced the dragon and we didn't die, so now we need to find some way to keep going with the knowledge that dragons exist. We take the knowledge and the feelings associated with the experience and we put them in a place that will minimize the amount of damage they can create.

We can put that experience into the superficial tissues of the Sinew channels. We can put it into the peripheral blood circulation of the Luo-collateral system, holding it in the limbs or in the vessels that are closer to the surface of the body. If need be, we can divert it into the joints through the Divergent channels, or we may dump it into the lower abdomen under the control of the Dai mai. This puts the dragon as far away from the heart as it can get.

This creation of latency needs to be maintained, so we use our resources of qi, blood, body fluids and essence to keep that pathogen, trauma or toxic experience away from the organs. This redirection of those resources then diverts the course of our curriculum. It changes how our genetics are expressed. It changes our beliefs about ourselves. We are not even aware that when we are resisting change, we are changing. We are becoming less of who we were meant to be. This type of change is not supporting our growth and development. Our resources are no longer being used for the evolution of our consciousness. The change is focused on survival. The longer we sustain this change through the creation and maintenance of latency, the more we deplete our resources. This depletion affects not only the post-natal resources we generate daily but also the pre-natal resources we were gifted to support our growth and development. This results in the creation of chronic, degenerative diseases that are less life-threatening but more life-altering.

This is the type of disease for which modern medicine has little to offer. The treatment for these conditions is typically focused on the amelioration of the symptoms that cause the most suffering, but this treatment does nothing for the underlying problem. It does little for the consumption of resources that are being used to maintain the latency. It does not deal with structural changes that occur over time. It cannot address the threat to the constitution. It may even devalue the complex relationship between body and mind that results in the rigid or fixated beliefs that come about during this process. I often hear stories from patients who are deeply suffering while the quality of their life is declining. They are told by the doctors that they turn to that there is nothing wrong with them, or if there is a diagnosis, that there is no effective treatment or cure. The focus of treatment is usually on the use of pharmaceuticals to minimize the damage or the perception of suffering, which, in some ways, is similar to creating latency. You have arthritis, take this NSAID and your pain will be diminished, so that you can keep using the joints. But what is the cost of the NSAID and how does continuing to use the joints, without understanding what brought you to this condition in the first place, serve you? Maybe the NSAIDs become a temporary measure that eases the suffering in the hopes that you will figure out what you need to do to change? But how many patients actually know that there is still work to be done? How many patients with chronic conditions know that they need to change their diet and lifestyle, and that doing so might actually turn around the disease process and lead them back to a state of good health? Even fewer know they need to examine their beliefs about themselves or their condition. How many know they need to deal with their response to their dragon? Do they realize that there may be a possibility that early trauma predisposed them to their current state of health?

The biggest cost of resistance and survival is the impact that it has on growth and development. If you look, for instance, at the process of addiction, what you see is an individual who experiences trauma that cannot be reconciled and so they look for something that distances themselves from the experience of that trauma. The substance of choice then creates a buffer that separates them, usually temporarily, from the feelings associated with that trauma. Over time, usage increases in frequency and decreases in effect, which leads to a cycle of self-destruction that ultimately results in death or, if they are lucky, awakening. Once this cycle begins, all resources are focused on the avoidance of feelings and awareness. They want to forget. This habituated state makes it impossible to use resources for growth. A 40-year-old man who started using at the age of 14 is, for all intents and purposes, still 14. If he is lucky enough to awaken instead of die, he will have to restart the process of growth, not from 40 but from 14. When we are maintaining latency, we are not growing.

We are presented with an opportunity every time a patient comes to us with a chronic condition that isn't responding to the standard of care. That opportunity is the ability to create an environment, through our treatments, that gives the patient the ability to step away from the dragon and assess the actual threat. We are capable, through the channel system, of engaging Wei, Ying and Yuan qi in a way that allows the patient to let go of that which is stored in latency and reclaim the sovereignty of Self. We can also provide the information through our treatments that allow the patient to restore the use of their Observer, more consciously and with intent. This intent can then lead to the ability to overcome reflex and habituation so they might choose differently. They can let go of their resistance and make a risk assessment that favors growth and development. Instead of housing and feeding the dragon, we can send the dragon away.

"Resistance is futile." For those of you who are sci-fi fans, you may have heard that phrase uttered by the Master, a renegade Time Lord in the *Doctor Who* series or maybe you heard it in the monotone voice of the Borg in *Star Trek*, before the act of complete assimilation. Either way, I do not think it is accurate. I don't think resistance is futile; I think resistance is inevitable. I think it is human nature to resist, but that resistance need not be a permanent state. Resistance isn't the problem. Perpetual resistance without consciousness is where we lose the capacity for thriving. Embrace your resistance as necessary to support survival but don't let it stop you from being all you are meant to be.

---- CHAPTER 3 ----

FIVE SPIRITS/WU SHEN

E ach of the five yin organs provides residence for a spirit or mental faculty. These spirits are expressions of the divine incarnated into our human form. The relationship between the five spirits encompasses the mental and spiritual aspects of humanity. They empower us to manifest our destiny instead of living a "fated" life. The five spirits allow us to change our lives through conscious intention. They are the active impulse that ignites our inborn potential. The five spirits are an important part of what makes each of us unique individuals. To move from surviving to thriving, we need the support of these five spirits. We need them healthy and harmonized. Spiritual alignment increases the possibility of physical, emotional and mental well-being. A healthy Shen is the basis of a positive prognosis for recovery.

THE PO: BREATH OF LIFE

In her poetry collection, *meant to wake up feeling* (2014), Aimee Herman says, "When they ask you how you're doing, tell them you're working on a master's degree on breath control." This is truly the work of the Po.

The Po/Corporeal Soul is the "spirit" that resides in the Lungs. It is a consolidating (centripetal) force that draws experience in. This aspect of spirit wants to be earthbound. It wants to have a full physical experience of what it means to exist contained in a body. It is the aspect of our spiritual essence that wants the pain, the pleasure, the variety of sensation that is possible in the human experience. This is the Pinocchio of souls. It doesn't want to be a wooden puppet. It wants to be a real boy with real feelings.

Through respiration, we are bringing the outside world in. When we breathe in, we are embracing the experience of living. We are asking to feel everything that goes with being embodied. When we are overwhelmed by that experience and we cannot process everything that is coming in, we stop breathing. Since we need to breathe to live, we stop breathing for a moment and then we reset the breath to survival mode. This mode of breathing is significantly shallower. We limit the amount coming in, and also the depth that it can enter. You can see this in children who are having a hard time with emotionally challenging experiences. Most toddlers are natural belly breathers. They are curious about the world and eager to bring the world in, but when they are very upset or overwhelmed, they will hold their breath. They will do that as long as possible, and then they will make their breath shallow by panting. This is the Corporeal Soul's attempt to modulate experience. They are overwhelmed by sensation, and when they breathe less, they "feel" less. This type of shallow breathing impacts oxygen uptake and puts the Wei qi on high alert, and self-soothing then becomes challenging. Anyone who has ever tried to calm a child having a meltdown will attest to the difficulty. It is only when they feel safe enough to return to that natural belly breathing that they will calm. One of the ways we do that for children is to hold them in a way that provides the sensations associated with safety. In doing this, we are using the function of the Po to down-regulate the Wei qi response.

The same is mostly true for adults. People who are under stress or uncomfortable with the sensations of living have learned to breathe for existence. The diaphragm constricts and breathing is restricted to the higher portions of the lungs. When we breathe this way, we are getting less oxygen but also less information. The reduction of oxygen unfortunately puts the Wei qi into a state of hypervigilance.

This hypervigilance may present as anxiety or being easily startled, or it may present as insomnia or digestive problems. Even as adults, we might find ourselves thinking, "I want my mommy or I need a hug." Instinctively, we know we need to feel safer. The difference between us and toddlers is that we are less likely to go back to the belly breathing because we have more knowledge of the world around us. Even if we get the hug, we are less likely to be able to hold on to that sense of safety and live in the world. The irony of it all is that the fix for this state of distress is...that's right, breathing.

There is a style of breathing that can be used to calm the nervous system down and bring the patient back into a more relaxed state. Many meditation practices focus on the breath for calming and there are various forms of this type of calming breath, but the key feature is an *exhale that is longer than the inhale*. This is said to down-regulate the "fight or flight" response of the sympathetic nervous system and up-regulate the "rest and digest" response of the parasympathetic nervous system. Seen more simply, when the Po is overwhelmed by taking too much in, we can breathe in a way that is more "out" than "in," thus limiting the input until we can regain ground. This type of breathing also helps us to "let go" of things that are holding us hostage and keeping us in the anxious state.

This process corresponds to the reptilian brain. The whole "stop breathing" thing is a reflexive response to the outside world. Patients do not do this consciously; in fact, they are usually unaware of how little they are breathing. Often, they don't recognize the diminished body sensation (numbing) that comes from holding the breath. It still surprises me how many patients are shocked to discover that they are unable to take a deep breath.

Because the Po is linked to the sinews through the Wei qi, the unconscious emotional response to being overwhelmed results in somatization of the emotions into the superficial tissues. This may be because we are better able to manage physical pain than emotional pain. When we correlate this process to the channel system, however, we see that anything that is somatized in the superficial tissues will be held far away from the organs, which will then increase the chances of survival. This is how body memory, bracing and armoring are created as a form of self-defense. In that sense, you can think of the Po as the somatic expression of the soul.

There are seven Po that are related to seven major categories of life lessons. We are not necessarily here to learn all seven but perhaps our curriculum requires that we learn three or maybe four. These lessons are offered to us as an opportunity to grow and become more of who we are. This is a chance to become more human so that when our life is over, we can transcend the body having done everything we can to have lived fully.

In each stage of life, a specific Po is active. As we learn the lesson of that Po, to the best of our abilities, we can release that Po as the next lesson (Po) arrives. If we experience trauma during the time when a Po is active, it can impede our ability to learn the lesson. This results in us getting stuck in the curriculum of that Po. Trauma impedes growth; it affects our ability to experience life fully.

The Po resides in the lungs and therefore is associated with the righteous nature of metal. The hardness of metal often impedes our neutrality, making the ability to learn from our experiences more challenging. If we are feeling righteous or superior in the face of the lesson to be learned, then we may suffer a disconnect from spirit that leads to a deep sense of loneliness. This experience of loneliness is amplified by shallow breathing. We resist the painful lesson and then we feel more disconnected from life and those around us. This separation causes the type of loneliness that you can feel in a crowded room. It has nothing to do with company and everything to do with being disconnected from life.

The Po provides physical movement for jing, making it responsible for physiological function. If the Po is impeded, then function suffers. When we forget to breathe, we are impeding our ability to function optimally. When the Po is functioning well, it takes in and retains that which has worth and releases that which has no worth. In the search for sensation, it is looking for value. The Po wants to benefit from being embodied. The struggle of the Po is this: *That which is most valuable is least substantial.* As human beings, we struggle to find peace and happiness, and we do that in many ways. We try to find the right job, the best home, the right partner. We are looking for substantial things that will make us happy. We are disappointed when we find that these things do not actually result in happiness. That which brings peace and happiness is least substantial. It's not about the stuff.

Acupuncture points to support the Po

UB-42/Po Hu: Outer-shu point of the Lungs

This point supports the ability of the Po to be fully embodied and live in the moment. Treats deep sadness, grief, worry or overwhelming mourning.

Ki-26/Yu Zhong: Front-shu point of Metal

It consolidates jing and blood in the chest to support the function of the Po and the virtues of Metal.

Lu-1/Zhong Fu: Front-mu point of the Lungs

Supports the Lungs' capacity to provide adequate residence for the Po. This point helps us manage our ability to take in and let go. It is useful for problems associated with bonding and attachment.

Lu-2/Yun Men

"Cloud Gate" is used to support the Lungs in letting go of old grief. I remember hearing Jeffrey Yuen say in class that, in some of the classics, Lu-2 was considered the front-mu point. To that end, I usually thread Lu-2 towards Lu-1. You know, just in case.

Lu-3/Tian Fu: Window of the Sky point

This point is used to treat spiritual issues or to support the release of Karma. It deals with issues related to the need for forgiveness. It is also quite useful in treating a deep sense of unworthiness.

You may also use any kidney point that anchors the breath and receives qi to support respiratory function. I like Ki-16.

Ki-16/Huang Shu

This point receives the qi from the Lungs and because of its location near the umbilicus is very helpful in grounding, centering and helping patients to become more embodied.

THE HUN: ASCENSION OF SPIRIT

The Hun/Ethereal Soul is more yang and less dense and substantive than the Po. This spirit gives movement to the Shen/mind. It provides the vision for directed movement including knowing when to advance and when to retreat, which is a function well used for survival purposes. The Hun is said to follow the Shen and resemble the Shen, but it is less integrated, more ephemeral. If the Shen loses consciousness, the Hun wanders. It is dependent on the Shen/consciousness to provide an anchor. As the spirit that resides in the Liver, it is the spirit of action that governs visionary states. It allows us to move freely in the world of thought, imagination, symbols and dreams.

The Liver stores blood when the body is at rest and the Hun resides in the Liver, so there is a deep connection between the Hun and Ying qi (the qi aspect of blood). The Hun helps us to balance and regulate our emotional experiences. It supports intuition and creativity and it aids our planning skills. It allows us to pursue meaning and purpose in a directed and creative way.

The Hun influences sleep and dreaming. This allows us to experience dreams as a way of processing experiences we have during that day that might be unfinished or unsatisfying.

When the Hun is unsettled, dreams may be disturbed or the sleep restless. When the Hun is agitated, it may decide to act. It might want to go for a walk and take you along with it. During sleep, we are typically in a deeply yin state; for many hours, the muscles of locomotion are physically paralyzed. Since the Hun is a yang spirit that supplies the impulse for directed movement, when it is agitated, sleep-walking or other parasomnias may disturb the sleep.

The Hun lives in the eyes during the day and in the Liver at night. When we are awake, it supports a vision of the future and the ability to move in the direction of that vision. At night, as it resides in the blood, it allows us to explore aspects of the psyche that are not easily available during waking hours.

The Hun is said to give us a connection to the collective experience and knowledge of all time. It allows us to drop into states that are subconscious, and in those states it gives us access to the collective unconscious. This may be why some people seem to know things that they have not yet learned or why some people have experiences consistent with the life of someone else. If you believe in past-life experiences, then perhaps you are experiencing the Hun's ability to connect you with something in that previous life's history that is necessary for your growth in this incarnation. If you are not a believer, then what might be described as a past-life experience might also be seen as the Hun's function of connecting us with knowledge beyond time. One could see this as the Hun allowing us to dip our spiritual toes into the pool of the collective unconscious in a purposeful way, in order to support our evolution. I have had what some might call past-life experiences. During meditative states or shamanic journeys, I have had distinct and vivid memories, which I know did not actually happen to me in this current body. Did I live this life in the past or am I somehow receiving the sensations and emotions of someone else's experience? It matters not to me, as long there is a benefit from those memories.

The elemental nature of the Liver is Wood. The movement of the Liver is upwards, like a seed sprouting, breaking the soil and rising upward, towards the sun. The Hun, like a tree or a flower, wants to rise towards the sun. As the spirit of the Liver, the Hun governs ascension and therefore might be considered the impulse for evolutionary change. An imbalance in the Hun can lead to the loss of creative impulse to grow spiritually. Or it may lead to the denial of the physical needs of the body in pursuit of spirituality or elevated mental states. There might be detachment from reality or logical thought or even domination of a single emotion which reflects an inflexibility in the Hun. The drive for spiritual growth must come from the place of being fully embodied. If it does not, it becomes a false pursuit, a sort of spiritual bypass. Of what use is a spiritual experience if it does not make you a better human being? What good is the "aha" moment of a peak spiritual experience if you cannot pay your bills or relate to your family in a loving manner? The bliss of spiritual experiencing is enticing, and it can expand your consciousness, but what good is that awakening if you cannot embody that consciousness to become more fully who you are? An anchored and well-nourished Hun provides what is needed for spiritual growth to be purposeful.

The inability to receive through dreams and symbols may lead to internal and external realities that don't match up with the needs or demands of the current situation. I once had a patient who at 42 years old wanted to maintain her fertility so that she could have children once she found the perfect partner. When she came to me, she was not dating, she was not employed, and she had not had her fertility assessed by a reproductive endocrinologist. She had dreams of having children but did not have a plan.

Acupuncture points to support the Hun
UB-47/Hun Men: Outer-shu of the Liver
This point roots the Hun, supports a connection to the collective consciousness, aids planning.

Ki-24/Ling Xu: Front-shu of Wood

Spirit Burial Ground helps us to let go of the past. Consolidates jing and blood in the chest for directed movement. It supports the function of Hun.

Hun She/Abode of the Hun

This extra point is located 1 cun from the umbilicus or 0.5 cun lateral to Ki-16. This point anchors the Hun and facilitates the "coming and going" of the Hun. It is on the pathway of the pre-natal Dai mai and provides a strong stabilizing and centering action for anchoring the Hun.

Lv-14/Qi Men: Front-mu of the Liver

Cycle Gate is about endings and beginnings. It helps the Hun set the pace or rhythm for life. As the last point of the Liver channel and the end of the Ying qi cycle, it is an ending that directs qi back to the beginning at Lu-1. We see this movement through the exit and entry points and also through the meridian clock.

THE YI: IDEATION, ATTENTION AND INTENTION

The Yi/thought, which is the spirit that resides in the Spleen, is responsible for our ability to think. It governs intellect and ideation. The Yi gives us the ability to generate ideas. It is active when we are learning something new because it governs applied thinking, studying and the ability to concentrate. The Yi allows for a mental response to experiences so that we can learn from them. Through its connection to the Spleen, it provides the context for experiences by banking the memory of those events so we can think about them and try to understand them. This is explicit memory, which is memory that is revealed by "intentional" recollection from a previous event or episode. It is not reflexive; we must choose to think about it. The Yi also supports the capacity for recognition. When we can recognize that new information is similar to what we have already experienced, this adds to the context and therefore supports learning.

The Yi supports attention and intention. If we can focus on something and give it our full attention, then it will be easier to learn. This spirit gives us the possibility of initiating change by creating intent. We place our attention on the problem and then we intend to change it.

The elemental association for the Yi is Earth. The Earth is the center of the wheel and it provides stability and grounding. As the center, it is in contact with the other elements, providing a stable pivot for movement. It also mediates seasonal transition by being a steadying force at the end of each season as it transitions to the next. This stability and mediation are location-dependent, as the organs of Earth, the Spleen and Stomach, are found in the middle of the body. It is also a function of intellect. It is our capacity for thinking that allows us to moderate our emotional experience and generate the ideas needed to survive or overcome chaos. It is our ability to focus our intention on what we want that initiates change. "Where the mind goes, the qi follows."

Ying qi supports this function. The ability of the Spleen and Stomach to generate Gu qi will provide the raw materials for the creation of blood. Producing the healthy post-natal resources of qi and blood is essential for memory and cognition. We need qi and blood to think. We need enough of it and we need it circulating. If you have ever seen anyone trapped in the midst of a hypoglycemic episode, then you have seen what happens when we cannot access qi and blood for cognition.

Let us now use the Yi to ponder what has happened to the digestions of our patients over the last 30–50 years. Let us think about the overuse of antibiotics (anti-life) that are cold in nature and destroy bacteria, both good and bad. Let us ponder what has happened to their ability to digest with the introduction of preservatives, chemical additives, pesticides and decreased water and air quality. Not to mention the depletion of the soil through big commercial agriculture.

Is it any wonder that there is a tremendous variety of diagnoses for digestive impairment? Research has now confirmed the impact on the brain and cognition of digestive conditions, even calling the "gut" the second brain. If our middle is weak, our capacity for thinking is impaired. This is not just about food; all experience is digested. To learn from our experiences, we must digest them and think about them. This is how context is created. To restore balance, we may need to "eat" less. This may be one of the reasons why it is a good idea to recommend vacations in nature. When we go out into nature, we can take in less of the chaos in our day-to-day lives, and what we take in is more nourishing. We need to do more than improve our diet by removing toxins and irritants. We need to detoxify our lives and find a way to take in less. We need to start thinking about digestion more globally and we need to change our "diet." Fortunately, we have the capacity to direct our intent towards that change, and the more we practice it, the stronger it will become. All we need do to begin is put our attention on the problem.

Acupuncture points to support the Yi
UB-49/Yi She: Back-shu point of the Spleen
This point supports memory and concentration. It may be used to resolve obsessive or self-destructive thinking. It supports the capacity for healthy ideation and the creation of context for learning.

Ki-23/Shen Feng: Front-shu point of Earth
Consolidates jing and blood in the chest to support the Yi for self-esteem, grounding and centering.

Lv-13/Zhang Men: Front-mu point of the Spleen
and Influential point of the zang organs
Helps eliminate unhealthy or obstructive boundaries, facilitates a healthy relationship between the Liver and the Spleen and Stomach

(stress, emotional regulation and assimilation). On the pathway of the Dai mai.

Ren-12/Zhong Wan, St-36/Zu San Li: Front-mu point of Stomach and He-sea point of Stomach channel
This is the primary triangle of the Earth School. It creates stability in the middle so that transformation and transportation are possible. Supports the Yi's function of mental clarity for learning.

THE ZHI: TENACITY AND DETERMINATION

The spirit of the Kidneys is the Zhi. This is usually translated as willpower or determination. I think of this spirit or mental faculty as being an expression of the fire of Ming Men. This spirit provides the drive needed for all the other spirits to persist over time. It gives us the ability to pursue a life-long goal with tenacity. The Hun gives us the capacity for directional movement, and the Zhi ensures that we have enough drive to stay on that path. Should we fall off the path, the Zhi gives us the drive to get back up and get back on track. The Yi gives us the capacity for intention; the Zhi makes sure that intention persists over time. The Po gives us the ability to "feel" life and, through the Lungs, the capacity to defend ourselves from the exterior. The Zhi provides the constitutional strength from the Kidneys to aid in respiration and ensure that we can continue to defend ourselves even when the onslaught is extended or overwhelming. It is the energy of persistence and the drive to survive.

The elemental nature of the Zhi is Water. As the kidneys have a consolidating function, so too does the Zhi. It has the capacity to store knowledge formed through the accumulation of thought. This impacts how wisdom is born. This consolidating function supports the stability created by the middle, which establishes a firmness that ensures the stability lasts. Like water, it endures and it may be seen as determination that is difficult to deter.

The Yi and Zhi are functionally quite different from the Po or Hun. They are less focused on experience or evolution and much more focused on staying alive. They are responsible for the maintenance of our pre-natal and post-natal resources. The primary functions of Yi and Zhi prevent us from depleting or dispersing ourselves in a way that can lead to "dis-ease." They provide the grounding and stability needed to survive the external realities that are creating evolutionary stress. This stability helps us to avoid emotional excesses by supporting the ability to think about what is happening to us. These spirits are stored in the organs (Spleen and Kidney) that are responsible for transformation, transportation and grounding. When there is an imbalance in the Yi and Zhi, we see cognition disorders such as confusion, disorientation, clouded thinking or diminished mental acuity. When they are weak, we see a disinclination to engage, resulting in apathy, lethargy and lassitude.

I see the functions of the Yi and Zhi as being related to the mammalian brain. Even though the Zhi, taking residence in the kidneys, has access to jing and Yuan qi, the mental faculty is very much about creating resilience and stamina in the interactive Ying qi functions of the other spirits. It is about maintaining the ability to think as a way of avoiding emotional excesses. It is about survival of the species. It may reside in the organs that provide the resources for the brain's higher function, but its function as a mental faculty is persistence.

Acupuncture points to support the Zhi
UB-52/Zhi Shi: Outer-shu of the Kidneys
Reinforces the Will.

Ki-22/Bu Lang: Front-shu of Water
Exit point where the Kidney connects to the Pericardium, connecting self-preservation to willpower.

GB-25/Jing Men: Front-mu of Kidney
Warms the Kidney yang to support the tenacity associated with Will.

Du-4/Ming Men
Warms and fortifies Kidney yang, supports will and delivers us from apathy.

THE SHEN: CONSCIOUSNESS THAT REFLECTS THE LIGHT OF SPIRIT

The last and arguably the most important of the five spirits is the Shen, which resides in the Heart. The Shen governs the relationship between all the five spirits and in doing so permits cohesion of the psyche and the emotions. This function allows for self-awareness. Though often translated as mind, it is sometimes called spirit and it represents consciousness. The consciousness of the Shen supports cognition, memory and the vitality of the five senses. When the Shen is healthy, memory will be accurate, cognition will be apparent, and the senses will be discerning. It is also responsible for the state of sleep. For restorative sleep to occur, the Shen must be settled. When sleep is peaceful and restorative, all the other functions of Shen will benefit. Sleep deprivation is a major cause of Shen disturbance.

The Shen is conferred by Heaven/Cosmos and is a direct manifestation of the will of that source. Our Shen is an emanation of the light of the Cosmos and is expressed in us as a luminous quality. The light of spirit can be seen in the eyes. It is the basis of our personality and represents our potential for true wisdom or divine universal consciousness.

Emotions originate in the Heart and the Shen governs our emotional life. It is aware of our emotions and develops consciousness from the emotional experience. Through this emotional journey, it gives us the opportunity to experience and cultivate, joy, compassion and unconditional love. To achieve this, we need the capacity for clear thought, insight, wisdom and an awareness of reality.

The Shen is the embodiment of all empirical knowledge, and this includes the distinct awareness of subject and object. In this, it allows us to engage the Observer. The Observer is not the thought; it is that which is aware of the thought. We are not our feelings or experiences. We are the awareness that is having those experiences. The Observer is beyond the reach of trauma and suffering, and viewing our experiences through the eyes of the Observer allows us to separate from the trauma and drama and see ourselves as emanations of spirit, untouched by tragedy. This consciousness is what allows us to forgive, to feel compassion and to recognize that we are all reflections of the divine. This is where we see the Yuan qi functions of the neo-cortex or human brain. Through the functions of Shen, we pursue the evolution of consciousness.

Acupuncture points to support the Shen
UB-44/Shen Tang: Outer-shu point of the Heart
Calms the Shen and instills the capacity for integrity and authenticity, especially in our communication.

Ki-25/Shen Cang: Front-shu point of Fire
Calms the Shen and supports the Shen's desire to let go and be liberated. Supports self-esteem and the desire to be fully engaged in living by consolidation of jing and blood in the chest.

Ren-14/Ju Que: Front-mu point of the Heart
Calms the Shen, regulates accumulation or stagnation in the chest (emotional constraint).

Ren-15/Jiu Wei: Luo point of Ren and
upper point of Bao Mai

Calms and nourishes Shen. Supports the relationship between all
five spirits. Connects Shen to Jing. As the upper point of the Bao
Mai, it restores the relationship between the Heart and Kidneys.

Our relationship to the five spirits is both alchemical and archetypal
in nature. From an alchemical perspective, we are driven by spirit
to pursue longevity and immortality. This is a deep desire for the
time it takes to transmute the profane to pure. We want to be better
people. We want to be the best version of ourselves. We also want to
leave a legacy when we go. This is about the rituals in our lives that
we create for the purpose of purification of the soul. Some turn to
religion to provide the rituals for purification. For instance, if we
were Catholic, we might ask a priest during confession to forgive us
our sins, and he might give us penance in the form of ritual prayer
to cleanse our souls. Others may embrace a traditional philosophy
or lifestyle that might involve the use of saunas, salt rooms, sweat
lodges or vision quests for purification. Still others might create
rituals around how and what they eat to create an opportunity
for purification. I also know people who are almost fanatical in
their protection of their exercise ritual. They know that exercising
regularly is what is maintaining their sanity and allowing them to
be the best version of themselves. It is important to assess how well
your rituals are working. The state of the five spirits can give you
excellent feedback in this regard.

Each spirit has an archetypal nature that is universally understood. The Hun is expressed in unique ways by each individual,
but the archetypal nature of the Hun as a reflection of the Wood
element is true for all. That archetypal nature is related to the
nature of the world and the Cosmos and the understanding of it
crosses cultures. It is commonly understood. If you draw a circle
with lines radiating outward from the edge of the circle, everyone
will recognize that as the Sun. It matters not that the Sun doesn't

really look like that. What matters is that we have a shared understanding of the Sun as a ball or sphere that radiates heat and light. We will all easily recognize the drawing. This is because it is an archetypal symbol.

We are by nature driven to understand this Universe and ourselves through practice. What we practice over time reveals the nature of the relationship between our Self and this archetypal nature of the Universe. Our dedication to a practice or discipline provides us with an opportunity to connect with the psyche at increasing levels of consciousness. As we practice over time, we become more and more aware of the synchronicity in our lives. The Universe aligns with us more deeply as we practice, and it sends us confirmation of that alignment in the form of symbols. For instance, we may begin to see the nature of Yi as a cosmic expression of Earth. Since food is an archetypal symbol for Earth, we might see this as a choice to remove sugar from our diet, so we can think more clearly. We might see it in the benefit of walking barefoot on the grass so that we might feel more grounded in relationship to the Earth. We might have a spiritual practice in which we pray to Gaia or Pachamama, in gratitude for the abundance that nature provides. Once we can see it for ourselves, then we can see the truth that connects us all. That is the nature of the archetypal experience.

We are reminded that what is archetypally true in nature can be expressed individually in countless different ways. One woman might express the archetype of motherhood by giving birth to a child. Another woman might express that archetype by writing a book. What is archetypal about the nature of motherhood is the ability to conceive of something, gestate it, labor over it, give birth to it, nurture it and then, in time, with unconditional love, let it go. It is not just the child that makes the mother. It is the embracing of an archetypal process or practice. This means that men can also wrestle symbolically with the archetype of motherhood. The archetypal nature of each of the five spirits can be examined through their elemental association. The Shen is associated with

Fire, the Po with Metal, the Hun with Wood, the Yi with Earth and the Zhi with Water.

The five spirits are vulnerable to pathological emotions. When we have challenges in life that produce emotions that linger, overwhelm, possess us or cause suffering, our spirits will become unbalanced. The Shen becomes disturbed and the Po, Hun, Yi and Zhi will become agitated. This injury leads to qi constraint, exhaustion of jing and damage to the organs. We have systems in place to release emotions that are considered pathogenic. If we cannot release, then we can trap the pathogenic emotions in areas far away from the vital organs, especially the Heart. Thus, once again, preserving organ function by creating latency is a means of survival. In fact, it is very common for a pathological emotional process, especially one related to trauma, to be the instigation for the creation of latency. Managing emotional states and the stress that might trigger those states is vital in terms of our ability to avoid latency or to be able to gather our resources to release latency. You may not be your emotions, but your emotions can derail your relationship to yourself. If this happens, you will indeed begin to believe that the emotional experience is the truth of who you are and then you will need to be reminded that at the core of who you are there exists a Self that is not damaged by traumatic experience. In other words, you will need to be made aware that you have forgotten who you are.

Because the writing of this book was completed during the Covid-19 pandemic of 2020, I am aware that we are all facing an archetypal challenge. We have had to face great loss and fear that required us to assess the manner in which we engaged our lives. We have had to learn a new way of being. This is not like flipping a switch or deciding to be different. It requires a lot of self-illumination and setting an intent to become more conscious and mindful. Once we set the intent, we must dedicate ourselves to that process, each and every day. This is one of the reasons why we need alignment of the five spirits.

CHAPTER 4

THE NUMBER NINE

The number "jiu" or nine is significant in the philosophies and practice of Chinese Medicine.

It is the last of the yang numbers in a base-10 system. It represents longevity and the emperor. It was a significant number in the imperial court and was represented frequently in the construction of temples and in ceremonial rituals.

In Chapter 7 of the *Miraculous Pivot*, there are nine types of needles and nine needling methods. There is a tonification technique called "setting the mountain on fire" that requires the practitioner to lift and thrust nine times. There are only nine points on both the Heart and Pericardium channels.

There are the nine palaces that are often represented in the Magic Square (3 x 3) where all the rows of three, horizontal, vertical and diagonal add up to 15.

4	9	2
3	5	7
8	1	6

Each of these squares represents a palace of knowledge or opportunity to gain experience.

There are many other cultural, religious and mathematical relationships to the number nine. It is well worth a Google search. You won't be disappointed. It is a significant number.

With all of this in mind, I have settled on nine recommendations for practitioners who want to treat patients stuck in survival mode. I hope that these insights will help practitioners avoid re-traumatizing a patient who is deeply entrenched in the resistance of survival.

1. THE PATIENT TAKES THE LEAD AND THE PRACTITIONER BRAKES

A patient caught in survival mode may be very unhappy or suffering from chronic illness or chronic pain. They may come to you to alleviate their suffering, but that does not mean they are ready to do the work needed to release latency or change how they relate to the world. I once treated a young and beautiful patient who, on her first visit, reported four chief complaints. They were, in order, anxiety, insomnia, addiction and wrinkles. When asked what she wanted to work on first, she was confused, so I asked her which of the four was causing the most suffering and she said...wrinkles. It would be easy to push that aside for what seems like more serious issues, but that would not empower the patient to take their healing in hand. It is hubris to believe that, as practitioners, we know what is best for a patient, but an honest, respectful and non-judgmental collaboration can set the stage for a very therapeutic relationship. It is a beautiful and effective thing to educate the patient, but ultimately the patient must decide what they want to work on.

Even when patients feel they are ready mentally or emotionally, they still may not have the resources or enough support to accomplish this. If they think they are ready and well supported, they may be in a hurry to get to the crux of the problem and get over it. My recommendation is this: The patient decides if they are ready or not, but the practitioner is responsible for setting and modifying the pace of treatment. We need to know when to put on the brakes. When you begin to release latency, patients often gain insight as to why they are in their current state. If that insight comes too quickly, it can be difficult to process. It is up to us to do what is needed to slow the pace. First do no harm. When patients are having difficulty with the process, we can do a few things: We can refer the patient to a therapist for more support. We can slow down the rate and dose of treatment by seeing the patient less often, or by using fewer needles or shortening the length of treatment time. We might also maintain the treatment schedule but alter the focus of the treatment to support the ability to process. I find Earth School treatments or treatments that focus on digestion very helpful for this.

2. RESPECT THE PAIN

When it comes to pain, the patient's perception is what matters. We do not get to decide what type of pain causes suffering in the patient. Nor do we get to decide if the pain is "real" or not. All pain is real to the patient suffering it. You can do your job and investigate the pain and what might be causing it. You might order X-rays or read MRI reports to try to understand what is happening to the body. You might also do a physical exam or ask about the patient's history, but you don't get to decide how painful that is. It is also ill-advised to compare one person's pain to another's. Everyone has a different tolerance for pain and suffering. Respect the pain as a way in which the psyche is trying to tell the patient and you that something is wrong.

3. THE ONLY DIFFERENCES BETWEEN PHYSICAL AND EMOTIONAL PAIN IS THE PATIENT'S AWARENESS AND COPING STYLE

When it comes to pain, patients have varying awareness about their pain and the nature of it. It may be very challenging to distinguish physical pain from emotional pain primarily because of two things. The first is that emotional distress can cause physical symptoms, and patients may not be aware of the emotional distress. They may have unconsciously somatized the emotion so that they need not feel it anymore, and the result is physical pain that can be easily separated from the emotion. The second is that some types of physical pain can cause emotional suffering, and some people may have learned to live with the physical pain, but if it lingers, they may have trouble with the emotional consequences. This kind of pain does not respond well to opiates but can be alleviated by treating the emotional distress. This is one of the reasons that pain management doctors often prescribe anti-anxiety drugs such as Ativan when the pain drugs are not working.

4. RECOGNIZE THAT RESISTANCE IS A COMBINATION OF HUMAN NATURE AND LEARNED BEHAVIOR

In general, people do not choose to resist treatment or healing. They do not choose to continue unhealthy behaviors because they don't really want to get better. They want to get better, but they are stuck in the reflexive responses of survival which make resistance the rule of the day. Not only are we all hard-wired to resist change, but over time we have learned or developed habituated behavior that has worked to keep us alive. That is predictable behavior, and even though it may impede healing or optimal health, it has served a purpose and we have come to count on it as producing predictable results. Better the devil you know. This is usually about a patient's ability to face the fear of the unknown.

5. SEE THE WHOLENESS

I have learned over time, as have many of my colleagues, that we cannot help every patient who is referred to us. Sometimes it is just not our work. When it comes to the kind of suffering that is caused by acts of self-preservation, I find that if I can see the wholeness in the patient, I can probably help them. That unbroken place at the core of Self is untouched by trauma. This place or aspect of Self remains whole, no matter what has occurred. This place can be seen in the eyes. It is the potential for the evolution of consciousness. Don't be afraid to treat anyone sent to you, but also remember that there is no shame or failure in knowing when to refer out.

6. YOU ARE INFLUENCED BY YOUR HISTORY, BUT YOU ARE NOT YOUR HISTORY

You are the person watching yourself being run by your history. If we can help patients to engage this Observer, then we can help them to create just enough distance for separation from the trauma. This gives a patient more agency and increases options for change. Many patients experience trauma or challenges in life, and over time if they cannot reconcile those experiences, then they will begin to identify with them. This identification makes letting go of the trauma or challenge almost impossible. We need to be reminded that we are not our trauma. We experienced a traumatic event. We are not our emotions. We felt them, but they are not us. This is particularly true when the impact of trauma reaches down to the level of Yuan qi. When the trauma lodges in the Yuan qi, it can easily impact our beliefs about ourselves and the world around us. It can also divert our path or mission.

7. LESS IS MORE

When treating patients suffering in this way, we need to recognize that they got to this point because they were unable to process everything that is happening in their lives. To help a patient like this, you need to give them information that is easy to digest. That means less information, but also it means a much clearer and simpler intent.

If we try to accomplish too much, too fast, then the patient will be overwhelmed. This is where the beauty of channel theory shines. Since the channel is doing the work, once we choose it, we need only reinforce the function of the channel. This can be done with very few points. We do not need to pick a point for every symptom because the channel itself will accomplish the job of bringing balance back.

8. EMPATHY AND COMPASSION DO NOT PRECLUDE GOOD BOUNDARIES

We can have empathy for the suffering that our patients are enduring, and we can have a desire to want to ease that suffering, but we must have intact boundaries to be most helpful. The distance created by healthy boundaries does not dampen our compassion. Boundaries provide the structure needed for our compassion to be a useful tool. In fact, good boundaries make it possible for both the patient and practitioner to feel safe enough to engage resistance. A lack of good boundaries can lead to chaos, which can manifest as manipulation, resentment, frustration and, even worse, co-dependency.

It is so easy to be invaded by the traumas of others. Practitioners must develop an empty heart that allows for the free flow of qi. To create a space where healing can occur, we must also develop detachment. If we become attached, we will suffer for our patients in a way that we can no longer serve them. We can and should have compassion for the suffering of our patients without being contaminated by the dark forces that hold that suffering in the very hearts of those whom we are attempting to help.

9. KNOW YOUR OWN RESISTANCE AND WORK ON IT

If we choose to help those who are victimized by trauma, then we would be wise to face our own "dark night of the soul." "Know thyself." Our own search for the truth is what helps us to provide an environment in which others can see their truth and be healed.

The more you know about your own resistance or defensive nature, the more you can choose how that resistance affects the therapeutic relationship. It is a little like knowing your biases. Everyone has biases. We develop certain beliefs about the way things are and then we seek information or experiences that support those beliefs. When you know your biases, you do not have to be run by them. You get to choose. The same is true for resistance. We all have it. The question is whether you are being run by yours. The more you know the nature of your resistance, the more choice you have about the impact that resistance will have. I have a resistance to feeling too much. For most of my childhood, I was criticized or teased for being too sensitive. To survive the judgment or ridicule of others, I have learned to distance myself from deep feelings, becoming less sentimental, more analytical, a little harder and colder. Patients can feel this, and they may interpret this act of self-preservation as disinterest, judgment or even anger. Because I am aware that I do this, I can usually see it quickly and then I can choose to stay in the openness or softness and vulnerability that makes for a more therapeutic relationship. This is not like flipping a switch. This is a life-long process. This is about each of us making an effort to become more of who we are and less of who we have become in order to survive.

Whether you choose to follow these recommendations or not, please remember that when you are dealing with patients who have created latency, you must do everything in your power to avoid re-traumatizing the patient. Do not let your honest desire to help your patient turn into an act of abuse.

---— CHAPTER 5 —---

THE SINEW CHANNELS

I have heard many therapists and self-empowerment teachers speak about the masks we humans wear. Over time, we learn to create a countenance or demeanor that is not a true reflection of who we are, but is actually a gradual alteration of our exterior. Changing how we appear on the outside changes how people interact with us. For many of us, this alteration in our sinews is an act of self-preservation. It is one of the many ways we protect ourselves from what is out there.

I remember a time in my early years of teaching when I was forced to look at my countenance and demeanor and the impact they had on others. One of my students passed me in the hall and gave me an envelope, and after an exchange of pleasantries, off he went. Inside the envelope was a card upon which was written a very sincere apology. This young man was apologizing for anything he had done that had made me angry with him. I was shocked because I was not angry with him at all. In fact, I could not remember a time in the classroom where I felt angry about anything he said or did. So, I wondered, why he would think I was so mad?

I wanted to think that he was misreading my demeanor. Maybe he was mistaking my passion for the subject matter or the intensity I felt about serving them well as anger or frustration? But the problem with that was my ever-increasing awareness that there were others in my classes who were also intimidated by me.

Our first layer of protection is in our sinews. Our Wei qi

responds unconsciously to external stimulus by flinching, ducking and dodging to avoid pain and injury. If the input continues and we cannot find a way to avoid it, then our sinews eventually brace for the onslaught of that input. This bracing can occur whether the onslaught is physical or emotional. It can even occur if the threat is imagined. In fact, the anticipation of pain and suffering is often worse than any actual insult.

I was braced against the judgment of my students. I was ready, unconsciously, to block out their disappointment and their anger rising from unmet expectations. I was ready to survive that because deep down I was afraid that I was not smart enough or not good enough to be standing up in front of them as a symbol of mastery and wisdom. That bracing made me look angry even when I wasn't. It was a sort of preemptive strike, and the energy it carried was loud and clear: "Don't hurt me or I will hurt you back." In part, those feelings may have had something to do with my lack of experience as a teacher. I was often worried about not being able to answer all the questions. But this bracing was also coming from a deeper place. I perceived a threat from my students, but the truth did not match my response. Even from the beginning of my teaching career, I was well loved and appreciated. Not by everyone, to be sure, but by most. I had no actual reason to be afraid. Where, then, did this unconscious reaction come from?

In my case, I believe it came from a very early feeling that I was not enough. I somehow had this internal drive that made me believe that I had to earn my right to be here. As the oldest of four, I took that responsibility very seriously. As a child, I did not realize that it was impossible to make everyone happy and that it was not my job to make it so. I always felt as if I was failing and that everyone's unhappiness was somehow my fault. I began at a very early age bracing against their impending disappointment. This was evident in my sinews, even in childhood. My shoulders were very rounded and I had an unreasonable amount of tension in my neck and upper back. I also developed a tension in my feet and the back of my legs that came from perching on the ground, like a bird on a branch who is ready to fly off at the first sign of danger. I often think about that curling of my toes as a way of holding my ground while someone was trying to pull the rug out from under me. If you add to the mix a few heartbreaks and a devastating loss or two, then you can see the development of armor so thick and so hard it could rival the Hulk.

I had learned over time how to protect myself, but the bracing came at a cost. With this angry demeanor, I lost the opportunity to connect deeply with my students and others. As I was protecting myself with this armor, I was also building a barrier to intimacy and the full expression of who I am. This defense made it very difficult for me to express the love and admiration I felt for my students and many others in my life.

I had a good upbringing with well-intentioned and loving parents, and still I built this armor. Now imagine a child who experiences trauma or the violence of war or repeated bullying at school. What might happen to the sinews of someone who hears "You're stupid," "You should smile more," "Nobody likes you," "What's wrong with you?" every day of their childhood? Imagine what might happen to the sinews of a child who is physically abused or sexually violated. Sometimes the memories of these threats are so emotionally devastating that we lock them away from our hearts on the surface of our bodies, in order to survive them. We somatize the emotional trauma because it is often easier to deal with the physical restriction in movement than the assault on our sense of Self.

Our sinews are a living and very physical representation of everything we have learned in order to stay alive. We have come by this pain and tension honestly, in a lifetime of heroic attempts to keep going. The price we have paid for that survival is an exterior that is unable to express the depth of who we are. It does not align with our inner truth; instead, it aligns with our basest fears. What would it be like to move more freely in the world? How would it feel to dance as if no one is judging? How would it feel to be truly in love with the physical abilities of your body and grateful for its survival skills? What would it be like to know the joy of authentic physical connection to another, where fear is not an impediment?

The sinews take on the responsibility of protecting us from harm. The more they do that, the more habituated and preemptive that protection becomes. These habituated postures and patterns of response in the sinews eventually lead to dis-ease. What was once a form of self-defense eventually becomes an unhelpful pattern that drains resources, restricts locomotion and results in impeded circulation. Chronic habituated holding in the sinews can result in joint and muscle problems, neuralgias, skin conditions and circulatory problems. These patterns can also eventually affect the organs they are trying to protect. We know that poor posture affects respiration and digestion, and tension in the sinews of the upper back and neck can make good sleep challenging. If we cannot get good sleep, then the organs eventually suffer. How we hold ourselves in the world has an impact on our health and well-being. The more freedom and flexibility we have in how we express ourselves physically, the more powerfully we can respond to the world around us. This does not mean that we all need to become contortionists. Some of us will never be incredibly flexible, but even if we are not, we need to be less habituated and defensive in our physicality and more aware of how and where we are holding on. If we are aware of when and where the tension occurs, we have a choice.

Wei qi, and with it the Sinew channels, will do all that it can to protect the body from trauma. Creating a defense against threats from the outside requires sufficient Wei qi that is circulating appropriately. Wei qi has to be able to adjust its response to differing levels of stress.

It's like having a security team guarding your home. That team needs to be healthy and well trained. You would expect them to be able to adapt and respond to any reasonable type of threat and you don't want to think about it. You just want them to do their job.

If they do their job well, you won't even know about the threat until after it happens—or maybe you won't ever know. Life will just go on.

The Wei qi engages the sinews and the cutaneous zones on the surface of the body to respond to as much stimulus as possible, assess the input, determine the threat level and then respond. It does this reflexively. You don't really need to think about how or why it functions. Thinking about it takes time, and time is of the essence when there is a threat.

Our grandparents and great-grandparents faced many more actual physical threats to survival than we do now. They faced war, smallpox, polio and unsafe workplaces. If we go back a few generations more, the lack of sanitation and good hygiene practices alone increased the physical threat to Wei qi. Unlike our great-grandparents, however, we have significantly more toxic sensory input to deal with every day. There is more noise pollution, air pollution and information pollution than ever. I live in a beach city just south of Los Angeles (LA) and, like LA, the only time it is ever truly dark is if there happens to be a disruption of electrical power. If you want to give your eyes a break from visual input, you need blackout curtains and eye pillows, and that is just one of the many ways the Wei qi is challenged. All of this constant input is quite overwhelming to Wei qi and we will find ways to buffer it. We can create a veil of dampness to act as a buffer. We do this by self-medicating with sugar, alcohol or recreational drugs. We also often turn to pharmaceuticals to buffer the input and our response to it. We also might try becoming hyper-focused on one thing in the hope of being able to ignore additional input, such as video games or binge-watching *Game of Thrones*. We are doing what we need to do in order to survive the input. We need to find ways to give the Wei qi a break. It is essential for the health of the Wei qi to find some activity or practice that helps it to let go of the defense for a moment and reset back to a healthy baseline of response. Or, more simply put, we need to find a way to relax. Perhaps we can commit ourselves to a digital detox. No news, no phone, no laptop for one day a week. For those of you breaking out in a cold sweat, maybe once a month would help. We could make a standing appointment for massage or acupuncture. Something like a sensory deprivation pod might give us the chance to reset. Nature can also be very soothing. We might sit in the shade of an old oak tree or float in the ocean. We need to find or create a place where we can let go.

Wei qi circulates on the exterior, warming all of the superficial tissues. Through the Sinew channels, it provides the capacity for locomotion. To actively engage the world around us, we need to be able to move. In addition to protecting us from trauma, the Sinew channels sustain our upright position, maintain our posture and govern our ability to explore the world around us. They do this by connecting muscles to bones and by maintaining the integrity of the structure. This is how you explore, but it is also how you duck, dodge, flinch, withdraw or retract in order to avoid injury. The stronger and more flexible your sinews, the more options you have in terms of response. Armoring as a defense may make you feel stronger, but you lose out on flexibility and range of motion. This armoring limits your options. When the sinews develop armoring as a form of defense, it changes your posture, your attitude and your perception of the world around you. It also alters how others perceive you. Acupuncture is very useful at freeing up the sinews and regulating Wei qi, and there are a number of forms of body work that also focus on freeing the soft tissues of the body, to alter posture and reduce armoring. Free the body, free the mind.

The Sinew channels are emotionally linked to the ephemeral nature of mood. If you are feeling something that is fleeting and you don't really know why you are feeling it, that is probably a Wei qi response. If you walk into a room and immediately want to leave because you feel uncomfortable, for no apparent reason, that is a Wei qi emotional response. When you respond to someone's emotional experience before they have told you what they are feeling, your Wei qi is responding and your sinews are already moving to protect you from harm. If you walk past someone on the street who is homeless and you reflexively divert your gaze, that is a Wei qi response. The Wei qi has determined that there is a threat even before knowing if the person is actually dangerous. That is because the perception of threat is not always physical. The Wei qi may respond because seeing someone who is homeless is emotionally uncomfortable. It determines that the best course of action is to look away. This is an active form of non-engagement that says, "If I can't see you, then I don't have to deal with the feelings that may arise if I acknowledge your existence." The Wei qi is trying to protect us from the suffering of others because if we focus on that suffering, we may be incapacitated or overwhelmed by it. If the Wei qi is balanced, nourished and flexible in its response, then perhaps we might respond to the suffering of others differently.

If we perceive the world as a hostile place, then our sinews will reflexively respond to that hostility. They might respond in a way that is defensive or perhaps even aggressive, because sometimes the best defense is a swift offense.

I have watched patients come into our office with that tension and hostility, and sometimes within seconds they will take a deep breath and you can watch the aggression fade away. They are responding to a changing environment through the sinews. I have also seen patients resist letting go, holding on to that defense because they do not yet feel safe. Sometimes this armoring is very deeply entrenched.

Los Angeles, I have always said, is an amazing place to learn but a challenging place to live. We are blessed with fantastic weather, wide-ranging diversity in culture and an abundance of resources. Well, except water—plenty of saltwater but not nearly enough potable water or rain. LA has a sort of interesting polarity that drives it. We have yoga studios on almost every corner, meditation classes, Tai chi and Qi gong being done in parks overlooking the ocean, kirtans and drum circles. We have easy access to food sources that allow us to eat organically or maintain a healthy vegan lifestyle, should we want to do that. We have a very large spiritual community that attracts amazing teachers/gurus. We have about everything we could need to maintain balance and pursue spiritual evolution... and we have Hollywood. Much of LA and its inhabitants are fascinated by youth and the illusion of external beauty. That is not the only downside of living in LA. The weather alone makes this place appealing to many, so we definitely have overcrowding. The traffic is outrageous and there is a lack of available and affordable housing. The cost of living is high, and don't even get me started on the dearth of parking. All first world problems for sure, but it is a stressful way to live. LA is a very competitive place. We are a city of strivers, and the perpetual companion of striving is failure. Not failure as a way to learn but failure as evidence of not measuring up.

Many Angelenos have temperaments that reflect the tension associated with living here. It is not unusual to see people who are angry, aggressive, anxious or depressed as a result of being burdened by the stress of trying to keep up. Not to mention the cost of being constantly surrounded by other angry or anxious people. In general, this city attracts people who are very image-conscious. We cannot let the world see how stressed we really are. We must present an image that reflects success. People are not supposed to be able to detect the pressure of living here. If you live here, you are supposed to be successful, "woke" and tanned! If you are not those things, then you must create the illusion of those things. That's what spray tans do. I am by no means judging spray tans or even the need to create an illusion. This is all a form of self-preservation. Wherever you live, there will be some reason to become defensive. We must accept this about ourselves and then start to recognize this reflexive response and decide more consciously if that response is serving us in the way that we wish to be served.

Over time, many people leave LA in search of a place that is less stressful or that simply has less input. Less traffic, less noise, less expectation. Those who stay, adapt. They develop a habitual or characteristic emotional response to their surroundings. There is no one specific character style associated with LA. It is a huge city and each individual has their own level of sensitivity to outside stimulus. Each of us responds in whatever way our Wei qi decides is essential to our survival.

If you haven't already done this, I urge you to look for this Wei qi defense wherever you live or work. Even in places where life is less stressful and more idyllic, there is still a response. I imagine that there are still places in the world where people are less armored and less defensive. I am also acutely aware of the fact that there are many places in the world that are much more stressful than LA. I know that the color of your skin and your gender have a potent impact on how you will perceive the world around you and therefore how your Wei qi will respond. There are places in the world where a higher state of vigilance is required to survive. That high state of vigilance is more intense and more common if you are a person of color.

Since it is often very difficult or even impossible to change the world around us, we may need to learn how to change our response to the world. If we can free up our sinews and bring awareness to our habituated responses, then perhaps we can alter how we are in the world.

I have always taken a sort of perverse interest in the tension created by the polarity of LA. It is an interesting place with a tremendous amount of diversity and opportunity to learn and grow. The older I get, the more I recognize the cost of that tension. Years of that defensive response can wear you down. I find myself longing for a place where the perpetual tension in my neck and shoulders might melt away and where the hypervigilance that fuels my awareness would be focused on birdsong and the sound of the wind in the trees.

These days, I am deeply and frequently pondering the impact of the forced isolation of the Coronavirus pandemic. I think about the physical effect of the virus on Wei qi and the Sinew channels. How will our sinews deal with the sudden need for masks and increased handwashing so that the virus cannot enter through Wei qi into the nose, eyes and mouth, eventually invading the lungs? I think about the fear we might feel leaving the house to get groceries or go for a walk, when we have no idea if those around us are infected or if we are already infected and asymptomatic. Does every little sneeze or cough initiate cascading thoughts that conclude with the possibility of us dying on a ventilator? I think about how braced we are, waiting for news about the infection or death of those we love. How much tension is created when we are trying to figure out how to pay our bills or when, if ever, we will go back to work? I think about the effect on the sinews and Wei qi when we watch the news all day or scroll through social media to get the latest updates, which usually focus on the disaster and very little on the success of treatment or patients overcoming the disease. Not enough good news to allow us to relax enough to release the fear. Will our sinews be locked down for six months, a year, a decade? Freeing the sinews is going to be a large part of our recovery process.

WEI QI AND PO

Wei qi is disseminated to the surface of the body through the dispersing function of the Lungs. This means that there is a strong connection between the Wei qi and the Po (Corporeal Soul) that takes residence in the Lungs. The Po wants to be earthbound. It wants to experience all that it means to live in a state of polarity. As the somatic expression of the soul, it wants to experience sensation. From the very first time we inflate our lungs, just moments after birth, we experience so much of what the world outside us has to offer. Do you know what was available to you at the moment of that first breath? Was your entry into the world gentle, kind and loving? Was it an assault to your senses? Was it fraught with fear and trauma? The very first time your Wei qi is activated, it begins to set a threshold of response that is attuned to survival and based on the sensory input. In some ways, you could say that the first breath sets the parameters of the autonomic nervous system. What will your brain perceive as a threat based on this early post-natal input? If that input is overwhelming, then the sinews will work to brace against further input. This is one of the reasons why infant massage has such a profound effect on a baby's nervous system. The sensations that the Po experiences during the massage send messages of comfort, safety and pleasure which may work to restore balance in the Wei qi. Unfortunately, that doesn't work with all infants. Sometimes babies, especially those born prematurely with underdeveloped lungs, may experience massage as too much additional input. They might even experience stroking, rubbing or patting as painful or distressing. For those babies, introduction to touch may need to begin with simple static contact or holding, like swaddling, which is intended to recreate the sensation of safety in the womb.

The Po is a yin spirit that is less refined than the Shen or Hun. Through inhalation, it is supposed to take in that which has worth and through exhalation let go of that which has no worth or that which no longer serves. One might say that it is the physical manifestation of spirit. It is that aspect of the soul that gives rise to sensation or, in other words, it allows us to have a somatic experience of life. With the increase in environmental input, the Po may be more easily overwhelmed. Aside from bracing the sinews as a way to deal with overwhelming experience, the Po is also responsible for the somatization of unconscious emotional experiences that are too overwhelming to process. Occasionally, this somatization is experienced as chronic pain or locked-down patterns of restricted motion associated with body memory. There may even be diminished sensation or areas of numbness, where unprocessed trauma or emotion is stored. One might also see excessive sensitivity in areas of storage, such as ticklishness or flinching upon contact.

Regardless of how this response arises, we are seeing an act of self-preservation. The Wei qi and sinews are unable to release that which no longer serves. In order to preserve organ function and ensure survival, the Wei qi traps the pathogenic experience in the superficial tissues (sinews) where it will be unable to interact directly with the organs. It is doing what it is meant to do, but the problem is that one of the reasons the Wei qi is unable to deal with challenging experiences is that it is constantly bombarded with non-essential and uncomfortable sensory input. Imagine what it would be like to try to defend yourself against a perceived threat while trapped in an environment that is uncomfortable in a number of different ways. Where is the actual threat?

How, then, can we help our patients to free their bodies and reset the reflexive nature of Wei qi so that it reflects a more conscious expression of Self? The Sinew channels offer us an opportunity to address this.

The Sinew channels are typically used to treat orthopedic or dermatological conditions. Since they circulate Wei qi on the surface of the body, we can regulate them to treat sprains, strains, joint pain, neuralgias and rashes. This pathology typically results in pain or other uncomfortable sensations, such as itching or burning in the superficial tissues. There are several factors involved in the pathogenesis of sinew conditions.

External factors

The surface of the body is vulnerable to pathogenic influence from exposure. Wind, cold, damp, heat, dryness and summer-heat can all become trapped in the sinews and cause disease. These exterior attacks often induce sinew symptoms such as muscle aches, joint pain, stiff neck, headaches and rashes.

Trauma

Physical trauma such as impact injuries or sprains and strains also disrupts the movement of Wei qi in the sinews, resulting in pain, swelling, bruising and loss of function. These are patterns associated with local qi and blood stasis.

Overuse or improper use

When we use specific sinews in an improper fashion or if we use them too much without sufficient rest, we can create a state of qi stagnation that often results in heat. Here we see common inflammatory conditions such as tennis elbow or carpal tunnel syndrome.

Organ pathology

Imbalances in the organs, especially those that are associated with Wei qi or the limbs, can result in pathology in the sinews. For instance, Liver blood deficiency can impact the muscles' ability to contract and relax appropriately, which results in cramping or twitching in the muscles. A lack of stomach yin can also affect the muscles, causing reduced tissue nutrition and increased inflammation, which over time can result in atrophy or Wei syndrome.

All of these pathogenic processes are readily treated through the Sinew channels. But in terms of self-defense, the Sinew channels can do more. It is possible to treat the sinews to support the release of armoring and resistance in the physical structure of the body. They can be used to treat body memory that is a result of both physical and emotional trauma. They can be used to unlock habitual, structural or postural patterns that impede flexibility of movement which may inhibit learning and growth. They can also be used to support shifts in mood. For this, it may be useful to look at the previous pathogenic factors with a slightly more expanded perspective.

External factors

If we take an expanded view of external factors, we can say that overwhelming or lingering toxic input can create armoring in the sinews. Anything you "take in" from the outside is going to pass through the senses and the surface of the body. That means sounds, smells, food and images that are not nourishing and supporting can all cause the sinews to go into survival mode and lockdown. We are in the age of information, and our ability to process all of that information has not kept up with the bombardment of stimuli. Our Wei qi is constantly assaulted. This assault may produce many of the same symptoms in the sinews as the external pathogenic factors. Wind-cold is not the only pathogenic influence that can cause a "pain in the neck."

Trauma

As physical trauma causes local qi and blood stagnation, so too can emotional trauma. It is possible to divert emotional experiences into the superficial tissues of the body to keep the impact of that trauma away from the Heart. This results in body memory that feels like physical pain or injury. Most, if not all, chronic pain has an emotional component. It is also well known that people suffering from chronic pain have a very high incidence of mood disorders that are likely associated with emotional trauma prior to their injury or experience of physical pain. The patient experiences the pain often without the recognition of its emotional source. All pain is real and physical when the patient is experiencing it, but if we as practitioners can recognize the emotional content, then we can help our patients to let go.

Overuse or improper use

When we overuse a part of our body, the sinews become habituated to that type of movement. The more habit, the less flexibility.

We come to rely on certain types of movement, which then requires us to brace in areas of the body to support the overuse. We can become very adept at bracing to support improper use. For instance, if you spend a lot of time at a computer taking in massive amounts of information, it is very challenging to sustain an upright position. We have a tendency to lean forward towards the screen. This then causes us to brace in the upper back and neck to compensate for the postural misalignment. One antidote to that is to get up and away from the screen regularly and move in a way that releases the bracing. We often find it very difficult to do that. Why is it so hard to remember to get up and away? In part, it may be because we are craving distraction. When we fall into the screen, we are not as aware of how we are feeling and what is around us. It is a form of tunnel vision that keeps us focused mostly on information that we are not really responsible for. It may be a way of avoiding the reality of our life. It might also be that the competitive nature of the world these days means that we must stay informed. Perhaps that heightened state of vigilance has become the new norm. This drives us, unconsciously, to be continually taking in more than we can process. After all, we do not want to be blindsided because we are not informed and aware. It is important for us to become more aware of our inability to stay present and aware of the impact of too much information. At what point do we turn off the screen? Regardless of the type of overuse, there is always a price to be paid for habituated movement. We can see the cost in the sinews.

Organ imbalances

People who have internal imbalances in the organ systems will do whatever they can to bring those systems back into balance. The interior of the body is vulnerable to emotional pathogens. If the interior of the body cannot restore balance, the prime directive of survival will force the body to minimize injury to the organs. This means that if the threat, which is likely emotional in nature, cannot be eliminated, it must be stored someplace that will limit its ability to negatively impact organ function. This is an example of the process of somatization.

Deficiencies in the organ systems may result in a lack of nutrition and circulation supplying the sinews. This may also make it very challenging to process emotional experiences, which then may result in sinew pathology. We might think of this as the sinews being affected by a Ying and Wei disharmony. The Sinew channels are not just responding to exterior input. They are also part of the process through which things are expressed or released into the world from the interior. That which is unable to be expressed or released may become "stuck" in the sinews.

To fully understand their impact and to determine how to release the Sinew channels, you must know where they go and what areas of the body they influence. The Sinew channels are grouped into yin and yang channels. The three hand yang channels (Small Intestine, Large Intestine and Triple Warmer) and the three foot yang channels (Urinary Bladder, Gall Bladder and Stomach) all meet in the region of the forehead and cheek. They are responsible for voluntary movement, gestures and facial expressions. The three hand yin channels (Lung, Pericardium and Heart) and the three foot yin channels (Spleen, Liver and Kidney) meet in the trunk and are responsible for postural alignment, autonomic muscle control, sphincter muscles and reflexive responses such as flinching, ducking and embracing.

Table 5.1 Sinew groupings

Yang/yin groups	Greater yang Greater yin	Lesser yang Terminal yin	Brightest yang Lesser yin
Three foot yang	Urinary Bladder	Gall Bladder	Stomach
Three hand yang	Small Intestine	Triple Warmer	Large Intestine
Three foot yin	Spleen	Liver	Kidney
Three hand yin	Lung	Pericardium	Heart

SINEW MEETING POINTS

Each Sinew channel has its own distinctive pathway and influence, but the three channels in a specific group overlap in a common area. Points in that area are called *meeting points* and they are a way to influence all three channels in a group with one point.

Table 5.2 Sinew channel meeting points

Three foot yang: Meet in the region of the cheek SI-18 or St-3	Three foot yin: Meet in the region of the genitals Ren-3 or Ren-4
Three hand yang: Meet in the region of the forehead St-8 or GB-13	Three hand yin: Meet in the thoracic region GB-22

It is not uncommon to see pathology in more than one Sinew channel at a time. A perfect example of that is sciatica. The restriction or pain in sciatica conditions begins in the low back (UB), radiates down into the buttocks (GB), and if it extends below the knee, it usually rotates inward towards the shin (St). The use of the meeting point in a treatment does two things: It can give you access to all three channels in the group, using fewer needles and creating one clear treatment principle; and if the pathology is limited to one or two channels in a group, the use of the meeting point may stop the encroachment of the pathogenic factor into the remaining channels. As we will see later in the chapter, meeting points are commonly added to a treatment to increase the efficacy.

THE SIX CUTANEOUS ZONES

The Six Cutaneous Zones are where it is easiest to see the armoring of Wei qi, especially the three yang zones. The Tai Yang zone covers most of the posterior aspect of the body. It governs the big muscles that are in the region of the Urinary Bladder and Small Intestine primary channels. This zone is much broader in area and influence than the Tai Yang primary channels, but it is also more superficial in its impact. You can see this as a sort of muscular extension of the Du mai. The movement is upright and moving forward with eyes looking straight ahead.

The Shao Yang zone covers the lateral aspects of the trunk, limbs and the retro-auricular region of the head. The movement is rotational and the peripheral vision opens. Shao Yang allows us to turn our heads and see our options. It also allows us to alter our course. Through the pivoting function of Shao Yang, we can be flexible in our movement and change directions.

The Yang Ming zone influences the large muscles of the abdomen and chest. It also governs the muscles of the face and the large locomotion muscles in the front of the legs. The movement here instills the capacity to slow down, to put on the brakes. These are the muscles we use to control how and when we sit down to rest. It is fairly easy for the practiced eye to see restrictions in these yang muscle groups because of the size of the zones. Restricted movement in these groups is not subtle.

The yin zones are a little harder to recognize in motion because they are smaller and on the inner surfaces of the body. We can see their impact more in demeanor or subtle responses to challenge or stress. In the yin sinews, we see the need for withdrawal as a means of survival. What we see is the "flight" function of the nervous system.

In the Tai Yin zone, the response to the world is uncomfortable and we start to retract or pull in towards the core. It is a bit like the beginning of looking for a way to hide from danger.

In the Shao Yin zone, we see the muscles of the medial aspect of the limbs contract and also the central muscles of the chest and throat. It is as if we are contracting so that we can limit input. We stop swallowing and we don't want to feel anymore. No more in, please.

The last of the three yin zones is Jue Yin. Its influence can be seen in the sinews of the hypochondriac region and the genitals. These sinews respond very strongly to fear and survival threats. These are the muscles that overlay the Pericardium loop and the Dai mai. Here the "flight" turns into "freeze." If you activate the Yin zones and their associated sinews, what you get is movement that resembles curling up into a fetal position. It is an attempt to look smaller, to disappear, to protect.

YANG SINEWS

The three foot yang channels (Urinary Bladder, Gall Bladder and Stomach) overlap on the face in the area of the cheek and they are responsible for how we physically explore the world around us. Their influence on the face can be seen in how the muscles of the face react to external experience. They also strongly influence the muscles in the pelvic region that allow for movement in the hips and sacrum. The leg sinews affect our ability to be grounded, braced in the pelvic region (girding of the loins) and move effectively in the world.

The three hand yang channels overlap on the forehead. They allow us to use the arms to reach out in the world, take what we want and hold on to it. Combined with the three foot yang channels, they control the muscles of the face that create facial expression. Facial expressions can either be a response to stimulus or an expression of our internal experience. Poker players look for the expression through these facial aspects of the yang sinews. They are looking for what is commonly called a "tell." Experienced players can read the sinews and determine whether or not their opponent is bluffing. Is your face an open book that is easy to read? Or do the sinews on the face hide who you are and what you are feeling? Do you have any control over that?

YIN SINEWS

Although significantly smaller than the yang sinews, the yin sinews are no less important. These sinews, which govern the medial aspects of the body, create stability and alignment by holding things in. The three foot yin sinews protect the genitals and lower abdomen, and they support structural alignment by influencing the arch of the foot. The three hand yin sinews allow us to bring the arms into the chest as an embrace or as an act of protection.

ASSESSING THE SINEWS

The yang sinews can be easily assessed through movement. There is an association between the type of movement that triggers or aggravates the pain and the six zones:

Tai Yang is active during extension and abduction, and the pain is aggravated by walking or driving. If there is arm pain, it will be worse with extension of the triceps muscles. Armoring in this zone gets in the way of moving forward in life. One will have difficulty extending oneself into life. It makes maintaining an upright posture challenging.

Shao Yang is active during rotation, and the pain is aggravated by turning or tilting the head and twisting the torso. If the arm is involved, then the pain will increase when rotating the arm while straight. Armoring in this system reduces flexibility and limits options.

Yang Ming is active during the process of stopping or slowing down, and the pain is aggravated by bearing weight, standing still and forward bending at the hips. If there is arm pain, it will be worse when gripping and holding with a straight arm. Armoring in this zone affects a person's ability to recognize the need to slow down. When movement slows or stops, the pain gets worse, so we override the signals that say we need to stop.

The yin sinews are smaller and can be assessed through movement, but they are also diagnosed through how we "hold" ourselves:

Tai Yin is active while retracting (drawing in towards yin) and the pain will be worse when the patient brings the knees to the chest or hands and feet towards the trunk. Armoring in this zone demonstrates tension in the sinews that are used to avoid emotional discomfort.

Shao Yin is active when the patient is performing activities that require rotation with a bent limb. There will be increased pain while pouring water from a jug or placing an ankle on the opposite knee. Armoring in this zone occurs when trying to connect the function and energies of Tai Yang with Shao Yin. The challenge comes with the misalignment between exterior (Tai Yang) and interior (Shao Yin). When the limb is bent, rotation is less supported by yang and requires greater rotation in the joint. The movement is less stable.

Jue Yin pathology involves a severe lack of movement with constant pain. This inhibited movement may make patients appear frozen or paralyzed. Armoring in this zone comes from that "deer in the headlights" kind of fear. We have withdrawn as far inward as we can and we are still in pain. We can suffer or we can get it. Once we are immobilized by this existential fear, we can remain this way until we die or we can have the "aha" moment that frees us from the fear.

Assessing these zones can help us to see where the patient is stuck. Then we can choose the appropriate sinew group to treat so that the Wei qi can be released. We also need to be sure that there is sufficient Wei qi to release the pathogen or stagnation. Pathology in the sinews is not easily resolved if the Wei qi is insufficient. Patients with deficiency in Wei qi may also experience weakness, numbness and a loss of sensitivity, with a low response to pain. There may be a need to support the underlying deficiency with moxa or tonic herbs.

The response is much different in patients who have an excess of Wei qi. Those patients tend to have an increased awareness of pain and high sensitivity to palpation and needle insertion. In excess states of Wei qi, the flow is impeded and one must correct the qi flow.

If you determine that there is more than one sinew involved, then they should be released in a specific order. Release the most interior first:

Jue Yin (Hand then Foot), Shao Yin (H-F), Tai Yin (H-F)

Hand yang channels: Yang Ming, Shao Yang, then Tai Yang

Foot yang channels: Yang Ming, Shao Yang, then Tai Yang

CREATING A SINEW CHANNEL TREATMENT

Once you have decided which sinew you are going to treat, you will need an approach that will support the freeing of the Wei qi. To that end, you might choose from the following point classifications:

Jing-well points: These are the most superficial points and they access Wei qi. Being at the ends of the fingers and toes means that they are located where the polarity changes from yin to yang and yang to yin. This makes them useful to treat wind conditions or initiating change in the sinews.

Sinew channel meeting points: The use of the meeting point associated with the sinew you have chosen to treat means that you can treat or protect the other two channels in the same group. For example, if you wish to treat the LI sinew for elbow pain, then you add St-8 or GB-13 to your treatment. This three hand yang meeting point allows you to broaden the influence on the muscles and tendons surrounding the joint to include those affected by the SJ and SI sinews. It also helps to prevent the pathogen from spreading to these other sinews.

The next aspect to consider in treatment is the modality you will use, in the area of blockage, to activate and release the stuck Wei qi. You can use tui na, massage, cupping, gua sha or plum-blossom needle. You might also use liniments (salves, pastes or plasters) that have an ingredient or two that rouses the Wei qi, increases surface circulation and opens the pores. Look for something with a diaphoretic or orifice-opening quality such as menthol or camphor. The goal is to revive or stimulate the Wei qi in the area of holding. This will help to relieve the pain but it is also useful if there is numbness or a disconnect from specific areas of the body.

If you like to keep things simple, then this may be enough. There are additional needles that may be helpful in reducing pain and restoring function. They are as follows:

Xi-cleft points are particularly useful for stagnation in the channel causing pain.

Shu-stream or Jing-river points can be added to your treatment if there is evidence of dampness.

He-sea points can be added for a number of reasons including cold-type pain, deficiency-type pain or dampness present due to digestive dysfunction.

If you are dealing with holding or pain in a muscle rather than a joint, then there are some additional considerations. It is important to address the "binding sites." These are the areas where the painful muscle attaches to the bones. In this way, you will be addressing the tendons and ligaments that are involved. You are basically choosing points that are above and below the injured area. For instance, if the pain is located in the muscles of the calf, then you might choose UB-40 and UB-60 as your binding sites.

Sinew channels have a much broader presentation than their associated primary channels. You need to restore function in the whole muscle involved. To do this, add points for the horizontal movement of qi. Using the calf as an example, once you have addressed the binding sites, then you need to palpate the lateral borders of the muscle for tenderness. You might find tenderness at GB-37 or St-40 on the lateral side and Sp-8 or Ki-9 on the medial side. You may also needle Ah Shi points for this function. It doesn't need to be an established point; it just needs to support the outer edges of the muscle involved.

You may also have to address any underlying deficiency that may prevent a healthy release of the pathogen. Wei qi is yang in nature, so if your patient has Kidney yang deficiency, then the Wei qi will be insufficient or unsupported. Points to fortify Kidney yang or moxa are advised. If your patient is suffering from Liver qi stagnation, then restoration of the patency of Liver qi is important. The movement of Liver qi supports the circulation of Wei qi on the surface of the body and in the sinews. If your patient has a lack of post-natal fluids supplied by the Stomach, then add points to nourish Stomach qi and yin. These fluids are essential for joint and muscle health. If there is pathology in the Lungs, this may prevent the dissemination of Wei qi to the surface. You may need to support the dispersing function of the Lungs.

The goal of sinew treatments, in terms of self-preservation, is to free up the Wei qi. When the Wei qi is released, patients will feel physically more comfortable and more relaxed. This will allow the Wei qi to reset its threshold of response out of "survival mode" and into "experiencing life" mode. Once the Wei qi is freed from whatever it was holding on to, resources used to maintain armoring are now available to be used in a more productive way. The release of Wei qi also allows us to express ourselves outwardly with greater ease. Building a wall keeps others out, but it also keeps us in. Once the wall comes down, we may feel more comfortable expressing our internal experiences.

Patients often experience what they describe as fatigue after a treatment. Freeing the sinews can indeed make someone aware of just exactly how tired they really are. Patients may also be confusing relaxation for fatigue. When you have been holding tension in your exterior for a very long time, you forget what it feels like to relax. It is also not uncommon for patients to feel a little vulnerable after a Sinew channel treatment. It is a little like cracking an eggshell. Once cracked, all the gooey goodness comes leaking out.

In their effort to protect us by keeping out what might be deemed dangerous, they both also keep things in. The tension created by the Wei qi and Sinew channels is a barrier that stops things from being expressed outwardly. That might mean they block full expression but it might also mean that the tension prevents things that need to go from getting out. When they are freed, the sinews allow for expression or letting go to occur.

I remind you that the tension is an act of self-preservation. It is deemed by the Wei qi as necessary for survival. This tension is part of a layered system, and it is wise to remember that when we see tension in the sinews; it does not mean that the sinews are the only place where latency is created. Acupuncture and massage can evoke an emotional release that is often unexpected by the patient. Once the sinews are freed up, the emotion is very suddenly able to surface and be expressed. Sometimes this feels good. Like a deep cleansing breath. We feel free of the burden of that emotion. Sometimes it is terrifying. The distress caused by this sudden release can trigger fear and the emotion might be recognized as a deep well of endless suffering.

A well-intended Sinew channel treatment can act like a steam-release valve. We can help patients to let go of the build-up of steam, at a pace that they can handle and appreciate. There are times when patients have deep trauma, pathogenic emotions or limiting beliefs that are running the show. If you go after those pathogens directly, before a patient is ready or before a patient has enough support, then the memories and emotions of the trauma will put up a fight and the patient will suffer. If you think of the Sinew channel treatment as an introduction, like a handshake, then you can use it to build trust with the patient. This says, "I see you and I am here to support you." We don't have to do this all in one treatment. We can "peel the onion" a little at a time and you can decide when you are ready to let go.

There is a kindness and respect that comes from the practitioner being able to resist the desire to go right to the deepest part of the pathology. We are not the ones doing the healing. Our part in the patient's journey is small and limited. We may provide the information that makes healing possible, but we are not with the patient every step of the way. We are not the ones who should decide how quickly this happens. Perhaps the greatest benefit of Sinew channel treatments is increased physical awareness. The increased body awareness allows the patient to move more effectively and defend themselves more appropriately.

When the Wei qi is circulating and well supplied, we feel more comfortable in our bodies. There is a sense of sovereignty in renewed occupation. We can now begin to develop a dialog with our physical beingness that increases the chance that we will hear the communication from the sinews before they need to scream in order to get our attention. We can, with this renewed freedom, build a healthier relationship with our bodies. After all, the Po wants us to be earthbound. Part of our destiny is to have a full human experience. We have the right to know the pleasure of sensation and to appreciate the communication of pain as a way of telling us that something is out of balance in our lives.

KEYS TO SELF-HELP FOR WEI QI AND THE SINEW CHANNELS

Although I am a big fan of getting help when we need it, I think it is also important for those of us who support people on their journey to well-being to empower our patients to take their healing into their own hands. One of the spectacular things about the practice of Chinese Medicine or East Asian Medicine is that it is a lifestyle medicine. We teach our patients how to adjust their lifestyle choices to promote better health.

So here are a few things that we can do to support our Wei qi and our Sinew channels in their ability to respond to the outside world in a way that is more productive.

Breathe

Wei qi is disseminated to the surface of the body and to the sinews by the Lungs. Breathing can alter our reflexive response to the world around us. When the Wei qi is overreacting to external stimuli, we know that the sympathetic nervous system goes into a state of fight, flight or freeze. We can down-regulate this response by breathing in a certain way. The important part of the exercise is to breathe in a way that the exhale is longer than the inhale. This type of breathing is very helpful for people with anxiety, panic and overwhelm.

Increase body awareness

When we have body awareness, we are less victimized by the habituated responses of Wei qi and the sinews. We can increase body awareness through forms of meditation called body-scanning. These can be guided or we can learn the technique and do it on our own. When we become more aware of where the tension is, we can breathe into and let it go if it is not serving us. Exercises or practices such as yoga, Pilates, Feldenkrais and the Alexander Technique can build our capacity for body awareness.

Reduce input

Remember that our Wei qi is responding to all external stimuli, whether we recognize it or not. If we can consciously reduce input, we will give our Wei qi a break. This may mean a digital detox or simply finding ways to create a moment or two every day where there is less input. A time out, if you will. A chance for the Wei qi to reset and the sinews to relax.

Embrace the natural world

Spending time in nature can be very healing. When we are surrounded by natural beauty, we have less unnatural input. We can find peace in a forest of old-growth trees or in a meadow of spring flowers. We can be soothed by the sound of water flowing in a creek or by the consistent rhythmic sound of ocean waves meeting the sand. We can align ourselves with the rhythm of nature and reset our nervous system to go with the flow.

Epsom salt soaks

Soaking your feet in Epsom salts (magnesium sulfate) supports grounding and relaxation of the sinews. Soak your whole body if you enjoy a warm bath, but I think putting the focus on your feet is more specific for sinew release and grounding. Since Wei qi is circulated by the Liver and disseminated to the surface through the Lungs, you can add a little lavender and peppermint oil to the soak.

Acupuncture helps, massage helps, sensory deprivation tanks help, but we must also make different choices. We must make changes in how we live our lives. We must make better decisions about what we let in and what we do to support our Wei qi and sinews.

A SINEWS CASE STUDY

To be honest, I do not have much of an orthopedic practice. Most of the patients I treat who have pain are typically suffering from the somatization of emotional trauma. For those patients, the pain is chronic, resistant to treatment and often more generalized and less specific to a group of sinews. Also, by the time patients are referred to me, the pathogen has usually moved more deeply into the system and latency has been created at multiple levels. Finding a case that is just a sinew issue for me is almost impossible.

For the sake of clarity, I would like to give you a picture of what a simple Sinew channel treatment would look like. These treatments are incredibly useful for acute musculo-skeletal injuries. If you treat athletic injuries, back pain from heavy lifting or neck pain from sleeping wrong, this system can be your new best friend.

Imagine if you will, a patient who steps off a curb wrong and twists their ankle. The ankle is red and swollen, and by the time you see them, there is already some bruising. The injury has affected the lateral aspect of the ankle. There is pain and tenderness upon light palpation and the bruising is visible from UB-60 along the Urinary Bladder channel and also along the Gall Bladder channel from GB-40 to GB-43. The three foot yang channels are the affected Sinew channels. Although there is no visible evidence that the Stomach Sinew is affected, it likely will be as the bruising and swelling spreads. To do a three foot yang Sinew channel treatment, you will need the meeting point. These Sinew channels meet in the area of the cheek so we can use St-3 or SI-18. You can also palpate the cheek area and use the most tender point. Using this point allows you to treat one Sinew and affect the rest of the Sinews in the group, and in this case, it helps to stop encroachment of the pathogen (qi and blood stasis) into the Stomach Sinew.

Next, you will need to bleed a jing-well point. This is very important as jing-well points are the most superficial points on the body and this connects them to Wei qi, the qi of the Sinew channels. The jing-well point is the way out for the pathogen. You can choose between UB-67 or GB-44. Much of that depends on where you find the worst bruising or swelling.

Now you need to treat the superficial area of injury. This can be done in a number of ways. You might use a "hit medicine" or liniment on the area of the bruising. You might place a plaster on the affected area. My favorite approach for something like this might result in me being accused of sadism but it is remarkably effective. I prefer to use a lancet on the area and poke a few holes. Yes, I know this is painful but I have never had anyone complain about the results of this treatment. It speeds the healing immensely. After bleeding, you can make a paste of Hong Hua and vinegar or egg-white and spread it liberally over the bruised area. If you do not have Hong Hua or a raw herb pharmacy, you can make a paste with Yunnan Baiyao instead. Once this is done, you can wrap the ankle, remove the meeting point and send the patient on their way. Or you can do more.

You could, for instance, add GB-34, the Influential point of tendons. You could also add GB-43; in this way, you are also addressing the areas above and below the injury. You could add Lv-3 or Ki-3. These points will give horizontal movement to the qi, which will increase local circulation. How much you do is really a function of how bad the injury is and how much your patient can take. These days, I seldom get the chance to do these types of treatment. They can be very satisfying as the effect is profound and immediate.

I am choosing Sinew channel treatments for different reasons these days. I am typically using them as a way of clearing the way for the deeper work. Free the body, free the mind. Like peeling the onion to get to the deeper layers. The case that follows is a good example of this because the Sinew channel treatment helped but it was an Eight Extraordinary Vessels (8 EV) treatment that finally did the job. I like to think that the Sinew channel treatment made some space in the sinews and lowered the resistance so that the 8 EV treatment could provide the necessary information for longer-lasting healing.

The patient was male, in his 50s, in very good health. He appeared physically fit, with an upright posture and good muscle tone. Although not particularly obvious, after sitting with him for some time I began to see the sort of "springboard" tension that is common in Wood types. He looked ready for action. He was gregarious in nature and his eyes were very clear and filled with evidence of good Shen. Aside from his chief complaint, the only other thing of note was a low-dose prescription for a statin drug, for cardiovascular health.

On his first visit, he told me that he had right-sided arm pain that he thought might be carpal tunnel syndrome. The onset of the pain was about three months before his first visit. The pain started after having surgery on his left great toe. He felt that the immobility, post-surgery, and the increased computer use during his downtime might be responsible for this pain. He also felt that maybe the pain might be coming from his neck, which was also affected by the increased computer time and lack of exercise.

When I asked him to describe the pain, he grabbed the muscles of his forearm just below his elbow and told me that the pain was an "ache" that was worse while shaking hands and gripping. He also mentioned that supporting those muscles of his forearm while gripping helped to ease the pain. Upon palpation, he had tender points along the Large Intestine channel from LI-9 up to LI-14. He also had tension, but not pain, along the Gall Bladder channel from LI-16, through GB-21 and up to GB-20. Palpation of the rest of the body confirmed the "springboard" tension common in Wood types. His demeanor was cheery and engaged. I enjoyed his company. He was lively and hopeful, and he had a good sense of humor. That demeanor was not quite consistent with the coiled tension in the rest of the body. He did not have spasm or pain in the rest of his body; it was just that his sinews were primed for movement, a little tense and ever so slightly overreactive. This was not glaringly obvious; it was subtle, more a feeling or an impulse.

His pulse was thin and wiry. Not quite thready. It seemed relatively consistent with his build and constitution. His tongue was very slightly paler than pink with very slight scallops and a thin white coat.

He reported being happily married and satisfied in his job and content with his life in general. No history of trauma beyond the surgery on his toe. He did not have the typical symptoms of carpal tunnel syndrome. I thought it was more likely that he had tendonitis, which was later confirmed by an MD. I also believe he had some postural tension in the neck that was adding to the arm pain.

I chose to treat his three hand yang Sinew channels. I saw the Large Intestine channel in this group as being the one most involved in the pain. The three hand yang Sinew channels overlap or meet in the region of the forehead and the meeting point chosen is usually either GB-13 or St-8. I chose GB-13 because of his tension along the Gall Bladder channel of his shoulder and neck. I bled LI-1, the jing-well point of Hand Yang Ming to access the Wei qi and release it. I needled LI-11, LI-10 and GB-20. This was all done on the right, which was the affected side.

To address his Woody constitution and to support circulation of qi and blood in the sinews, especially the arms, I added GB-34 and GB21 bilaterally. GB-34 is the Influential point of sinews and GB-21 opens the circulation into the arms and down to the jing-well points of the hands. Once the needles were in place, I used a moxa stick to heat the area around LI-10 and LI-11 until the skin was red and a little sweaty. Bringing the sweat to the surface helps to expel pathogens from the sinews.

This treatment reduced the pain by only 25–30% but the improvement was sustained all week. Because the relief was sustained, I knew the treatment was the correct choice. Because the improvement was only 25–30%, I knew there was something deeper involved. I then looked more seriously at the reactive tension and the fact that the pain in the arm began during a period of forced immobility after the foot surgery. This patient had no obvious reasons to create this tension as an act of self-preservation. He did not seem particularly traumatized by the surgery or the subsequent immobility. Still there was something there that was defensive even if that was not clear from his demeanor or history. I began to look at that as an imbalance between the forward movement of Tai Yang—"What's next?"—and the slowing down and braking of Yang Ming. Because of this and the reactive tension, I decided to do a Yang Qiao treatment.

This treatment was done prone, so I could address his back and neck. I began with UB-62, the master point of the Yang Qiao and UB-59, the xi-cleft point of the Yang Qiao on the right. Added to that in the following order, Du-9, GB-21, GB-20, Du-16 with the Gall Bladder points done bilaterally. Then, finally, to open the arm, SI-11 and SI-10 on the right.

Du-9 was chosen to open the diaphragm, ease the Pericardium loop and soften the Liver and Gall Bladder. Du-16 was added to ease the tension in the neck and influence the brain and central nervous system. This may ease the reactive response so that he can relax.

This treatment resulted in a significant reduction in pain even when he used the computer or became more physically active. He started to notice that the pain was moving distally towards the fingertips.

When the patient arrived for the third treatment, he was doing so much better that he thought he just wanted to reinforce what had already happened. He wanted to optimize the relief. He could still initiate the pain by forcefully gripping and shaking hands but he had to work harder to get a response. As the pain decreased, he started to notice a little numbness in his fingertips, especially the index and middle fingers.

I wanted to continue to work with the Yang Qiao but I still felt some points of tenderness in the Large Intestine channel. I treated the Yang Qiao supine so that I could easily treat the affected arm at the same time. In a sense, I was treating the Large Intestine sinew at the same time as the Yang Qiao. The treatment was as follows:

Left-side UB-62, master point of Yang Qiao and UB-59, xi-cleft point of Yang Qiao.

Right-side LI-4, LI-10, LI-15, GB-12 (point of tenderness).

Left-side GB-21.

Right-side SI-3 was added as the couple point of the Yang Qiao to reinforce circulation in the neck and influence the spine for the numbness in the fingers.

After this treatment, the pain was mostly gone and the subsequent treatments were only done to reinforce the progress and because the patient's insurance covered the cost of the treatments he had come to enjoy. I saw him a few more times for maintenance.

I think that his Sinew channel problem was complicated by this reactive tension in his body. He might have managed to treat his arm pain with a little physical therapy or maybe even just laying off the computer for a few days, but this tension he was unconsciously carrying slowed the healing. Once the Yang Qiao was regulated, he was carrying less tension. His Wood nature was still present but it was more relaxed and less reactive.

WHY CHOOSE A SINEW CHANNEL TREATMENT?

When we think about using a Sinew channel treatment for physical conditions, we are usually thinking about acute sprains and strains or neuralgias. Sinew channel treatments are very commonly done for sports injuries or overuse injuries, such as a torn rotator cuff or carpal tunnel syndrome.

For acts of self-preservation, the problem need not be acute and it most often isn't. Habituated responses that lead to armoring take time to develop. How do we then recognize the effect of these acts on the sinews? Aside from the typical physical symptoms, patients with Sinew channel pathology may have any of the following:

- Bracing or armoring in a group of muscles or specific area of the body.

- Defensive response to palpation, such as ticklishness or flinching, that is often indicative of body memory.

- Hypervigilance, startle reflex or overreaction to exterior stimuli.

- Hypersensitivity to sensory input (smells, sounds, light).

- Any physical condition that restricts movement.

- If the patient's reflexive response to requests is "No" first (perceived threat managed by avoidance).

- If people think they know you but they don't, or if what you portray on the outside in terms of demeanor or facial expression does not elicit the response you hoped for. I put "resting bitch face" in this category, especially if you are not aware that you have it.

It is important to remember that the whole channel system is interconnected. The Sinew channels and all the other secondary vessels are extensions of the Primary channels. An insult on one system will eventually affect another. Just because a person has sinew pathology does not mean they are pathology-free elsewhere. It also does not mean that the root of a particular problem and its manifestation are in the same level of qi. For instance, one could have a Sinew channel issue in the three hand yin sinews, that is causing pain that might be diagnosed as carpal tunnel syndrome, but the root of that pain may not be too much time at the computer. The root of the pain may be a somatization of emotion from childhood trauma or it may come from being overwhelmed by life's challenges and trying to hold on too tight.

As the person creating the space for healing to occur and as the one responsible for providing information to facilitate that healing, you must decide where to begin. Do you treat the symptom? Do you treat the root? Is it possible to treat both at the same time? Deciding to do a Sinew channel treatment means that you have recognized the benefit or necessity of treating the outside first. You have discerned that freeing the exterior is a good place to begin.

CHAPTER 6

THE LUO-COLLATERAL SYSTEM

YING QI: DIGESTION, EMOTION AND INTERACTION

Ying qi (nutritive qi) is the qi aspect of blood. This function of qi circulates in the interior and as it resides in the blood it is responsible for providing nourishment to the body. This ability to nourish depends on digestion. This is not just about what we eat or how we eat it. The environment in which we eat also affects our ability to be nourished. Whole and healthy foods, eaten in an environment that is fraught with conflict, are much less nourishing than foods eaten in an environment that supports relaxation, harmony and pleasure.

To go a step further, every experience you have in life is something your Ying qi will attempt to digest or "internalize." When you think about digestion, think more broadly than food. This is about our ability to digest life and from that digestive process find something that is nourishing to the body, mind and spirit. Ying qi governs this process of internalization. How much are you "taking in" and can you digest it all?

Certainly, diet is a large part of that. Are you eating well? Do you have foods in your diet that nourish your body, mind and spirit? Can you easily digest these foods, or do you struggle with some of them? Perhaps you can digest the foods that feed your body, but you have more difficulty with the foods that feed your soul. Maybe you are comforted by foods or experiences that feed the soul but have more trouble digesting the foods that feed your body. How many people do you know that have food sensitivities? This reaction, to that which might in others be considered nourishing, provokes a response that is uncomfortable, unpleasant and a rejection of nourishment.

Add to that the news of the world, social media, your relationships with friends and family, your job, your co-workers and your neighbors. All interaction and input will need to be digested. Experiences associated with all of this pass through the buffer of Wei qi and engage Ying qi. Ying qi is then required to internalize or reject the experiences in a way that ultimately is supposed to provide nourishment. This post-natal nourishment keeps us going each day and it also supports our pre-natal resources. A portion of the qi we produce from the resources we take in is stored in the Kidneys as jing. This means that what we digest or internalize may be used to help us to fulfill our curriculum. If we do not have access to enough nourishment, then we will begin to drain our pre-natal resources sooner than we should. Unless we have been gifted with an abundance of pre-natal resources, this may leave us too weakened or distracted to stay on course for a life of meaning and purpose.

When patients have "digestive" symptoms, you need to look at what they are eating and how they are eating it, and then you need to look beyond food to what other things they are trying to digest. Are they nauseous because they ate too much or is their symptom occurring because they watch the news while they are eating? Are they struggling to internalize the endless continuation of violence that is evidenced by the ever-increasing incidence of mass shootings? Do they have heartburn because they have a problem with too many spices or fatty foods, or are they struggling to process the fear, anxiety or worry that arises every day when their social media hammers on about how the people they entrust to lead them are failing or, worse, abandoning them? Are they able to find nourishment in anything they internalize? Can they reject the toxic input, or at the very least can they balance the toxic input with enough nourishment from other sources? All of this is supported by the functions of Ying qi.

It's all qi. We are speaking now of the internalization process of Ying qi as if that is separate from Wei qi. But anything that comes from the outside, like food, must pass through Wei qi to get to Ying qi. By the time it reaches Ying qi, the Wei qi has either allowed it in or failed to get rid of it. Therefore, many pathological processes of digestion such as food sensitivities may be considered a lack of harmony between Ying and Wei. We need to find ways to slow the input from the outside, to give the inside more time to digest. Our digestion may need us to find ways to help our Wei qi set stronger boundaries about what we allow in. It is not surprising than many modern diseases are failures in digestion. Leaky gut and small intestine bacterial overgrowth (SIBO) are just a couple of examples of how the Wei qi in the Fu organs is overwhelmed. This failure in the Wei qi then allows pathogens access to the interior, and our ability to nourish ourselves is impaired. This disharmony of Ying and Wei negatively impacts our ability to think clearly and choose well. The gut is considered a second brain. Disruption of Ying and Wei, in the digestive tract, can affect both our cognition and our nervous system. We need to find ways to support "digestive" function by altering our diet or improving our elimination through the Fu organs. We need to examine what we take in and how well we let go. This will help us to find a balance between Ying and Wei.

The internal terrain of Ying qi is the dwelling place of our emotional experience. Emotions at this level are targeted and specific, and we are usually aware of what triggers them. For example, at my age I like to think that I have finally let go of many of those things that used to send my red-headed younger self into a fit of rage. However, on the days when I have to get on the highway, I still might find myself quite comically triggered into frustration and anger by those, shall we say, casual drivers, who are completely unaware that the fast lane is for passing slower traffic. You know those drivers. They are the ones who are in that lane, going the speed limit or slower, while dozens of cars are piled up behind them waiting for them to get out of the way. It used to anger me even further if, for some reason, I got the sense that they are trying to police traffic. Clearly, I have issues with people slowing me down, deciding what is best for me, and also those who are unconscious of the effect they are having on others. It was not about wanting to go faster, it was more about being impeded, held back. In earlier times, as the expletives would spew out of my mouth like an erupting volcano, my son would say to me, "Mom, you know they can't hear you, right?" He was clearly not triggered by the same experience. These Ying qi responses or emotional interludes have little to do with being present in the moment. They are typically triggered because we have cataloged other similar experiences from our past and we are responding emotionally to those memories. It is not about the casual drivers; it is about what they represent to me.

This qi is about choice, especially lifestyle choices. As it is more conscious than Wei qi, it allows for the possibility that we can understand why we do what we do. In that sense, it is about learning from our experiences. We hold the memory of our experiences in the blood. This holding function allows us to create context for each experience by cataloging them so that we can compare them to current experiences. If we can hold on to the memories of the emotions or judgments of uncomfortable experiences, then it is easier to avoid making choices that recreate them. If you can remember how embarrassing an experience was, then it is likely you will avoid making the choices that will put you there again. This process is very closely related to the functions of the Spleen, Heart and Pericardium. Generating the blood and holding it in the vessels depends on the Spleen's ability to transform and transport the food we eat and the experiences we have in a way that creates a context that supports learning. The spirit of the Spleen, the Yi, allows us to focus our attention on something in a way that we can intend for it to be different. Attention and intention give us the possibility of choice.

The Heart's part in this is to maintain sovereignty in the face of life's experiences. It does this in two ways. First, it houses the Shen-Spirit-Mind which supports consciousness. Second, it dominates the blood. The circulation of blood and qi is required for transformation. Stagnation of qi and blood inhibits growth. The Heart embodies those experiences that it finds supportive for the evolution of consciousness. If it is overwhelmed by experience, then it may abdicate the throne, allowing the emotions of our experiences to take over and possess the crown. We may then be run by our anxiety, fear or worry, forever stuck in an emotional loop like a hamster on a wheel. Constantly moving but getting nowhere. This loop can be easily seen in patterns of disharmony between the Heart and Spleen. Patients who have this disharmony are prone to rumination and overthinking, which then makes them vulnerable to emotional states that are irrational and will further feed the rumination.

The Pericardium has the challenging job of protecting the Heart so that it can maintain its sovereignty. A difficult job to be sure, especially in the face of the emotionally triggering experiences we face these days. Access to what is happening all over the world is available to us at the touch of a button, and we are also constantly exposed to the emotional responses of millions of others. One might hope that we can develop compassion and empathy from all of this easily accessed information. Most often, however, it is just too much for us to receive and digest. The Pericardium is the protective boundary of the Heart and if it determines that an experience is too painful, confusing or overwhelming for the Heart, it will reinforce the protective barrier by constricting the chest, in the hopes of keeping that experience at bay. The tension in that barrier is meant to be flexible and adjustable. It is meant to open the way to the Heart when the information is necessary for evolution and close the way when the threat is too great. The problem is that the overwhelming access to information and experience is so great these days that the Pericardium needs a bigger staff to handle the increase in information. When life is too much, the Pericardium tends to go into lockdown. This may protect the Heart, but it does not adequately allow the Heart access to that which would support consciousness. This constriction in the chest impairs circulation. If the Ying qi cannot circulate, nourishment cannot be adequately distributed, and transformation becomes more challenging. If we cannot nourish ourselves, we cannot support our own growth.

The functions of Ying qi can be seen in our capacity for relationship. If our Ying qi is healthy, sufficient and circulating well, then we can choose to be more aware of our emotions and the consequences of our actions. We will be able to consider the effect that our emotions have on others. Ying qi allows us an opportunity to think about conformity, responsibility, morality and finding a way to fit in. If we intend to be accepted socially, it may be necessary to repress or suppress some aspects of our selves or our feelings. Many of us are already doing this at holiday dinners when we are surrounded by family that we do not see very often. As adults, we are living our own lives and having different experiences from the rest of our family. This means we may have different beliefs or that our values, which are shaped by our experiences, may be different from those of our siblings or parents. We may decide to hold back from sharing our deeper thoughts and opinions so that the family dinner can be a more pleasant experience. For instance, my political leanings are much less conservative than those of most of my family. If I were to share my beliefs or fight for a particular point of view, this might cause distress. Since I also believe that everyone is entitled to their opinion and I love my family, I tend not to speak about politics or religion during the holidays. The tension that is created by these conversations is counter-productive and not well aligned with the spirit of the holiday. I am temporarily suppressing my expression so that I can enjoy their company. We can love our families and not agree with them. Some families are lucky enough to have healthier Ying qi that allows for discussions that are lively and educational and don't lead to someone drinking too much, breaking something or starting a brawl. Others are not so lucky. It is my experience that when we return to our families as adults, we immediately regress to the age of 12, and the struggle is to remember to be an adult, not a rebellious tween. It is the act of an adult to consider the feelings of others. We need not abdicate our beliefs for the sake of others but we also don't need to force others to alter their beliefs. If civil discourse is a possibility, you are most fortunate. But if discussions like these create suffering, then they are best left for other times. Healthy Ying qi allows us to model compassion and understanding in a way that demonstrates unconditional love or, at the very least, empathy.

It is natural for us to want to fit in. We want to feel connected to others. If we cannot fit in, then maybe we will need to find a place or tribe that allows us to be more fully who we are without judgment. This is a battle between an individual's identity and a collective or cultural identity. It is about social pressure and our relationship to the collective. This is about behaving in a way that is expected, depending upon the society in which you live. For example, in some cultures slurping your noodles or belching after a meal is expected, but in others it is considered quite rude. In the simplest sense, it is about learning how to behave in a way that is socially acceptable so that you can participate in all the benefits of society. It means that if you pass gas in an elevator (which by the way, in my opinion, you should never do), you are required to apologize for that breach of etiquette and hope that the people in the elevator will not judge you too harshly. What does someone typically do in this circumstance? Come on, you know the answer to this. They look around as if someone else did it. That is because they do not want to be recognized as the person who did something that is socially unacceptable. Even if they do it on purpose to enjoy the discomfort of others, they still don't want to be caught.

What happens when the family or society you were born into is intolerant or has restrictive values on what is acceptable behavior? What if who you are, what you want to do or how you feel is anathema to the society in which you live? I am reminded that in the USA, women are constantly in danger of losing their reproductive choice to a society that believes the decisions they make about their bodies should be controlled by those who have never experienced life as they have. How is it even possible that women will be able to digest the fact that their uterus, during its reproductive years, is subject to the judgment and control of people who, typically, don't even have a uterus? That this judgment is coming from some of the very same people who are now insisting that wearing a mask to reduce the spread of Covid-19 is somehow an infringement of their right to body autonomy is hypocritical in the extreme. Can you imagine what feelings a woman must suppress when she finds herself unhappily impregnated, maybe even against her will? How does one imagine what she might feel if she is told that she has no choice and must have the baby? She has a terribly difficult decision to make about how she will survive this, and she will be making it without the support or understanding of the society or family that is supposed to care for her. How can she possibly digest that without creating latency for self-preservation?

I also think about those in the LGBTQ community and how long they have had to struggle to find acceptance in the world. Many of them have had to sacrifice who they are or how they want to be in the world, for the sake of fitting in. No, it is very much worse than that. Many of our brothers and sisters have had to suppress the truth of who they are and how they feel to survive. To avoid the violence and judgment of others, they have had to suppress or deny their truth. I am amazed and inspired by those who have found the strength to intend to rise above the judgment of others to be more fully who they are. In our evolution as human beings, we need to be able to recognize and respect the sacrifice required to accomplish this. What does someone have to give up when they choose a path that allows them to express the truth of who they are? Do they have to give up family, friends, a job, the ability to have children, or do they even have to risk their lives to be who they are? The deeply emotional experience of being rejected for who you are is impossible to accept and digest without creating some latency for survival. If you had to face this, maybe you would be lucky enough to have people around you who love you unconditionally. Maybe you would be lucky enough that your family of birth would accept you wholeheartedly. But if you are not, maybe survival doesn't hold the same value anymore. The instinct for survival will continue to push toxic experiences and the emotions associated with them deeper and deeper. Eventually, Ying qi is overwhelmed and the problem is moved through the Luo-collateral system from Ying qi into the Yuan qi level and the constitution. How much rejection, judgment, violence, scorn, ridicule and ignorance can a human being digest before they decide to give up? How much intolerance can a person experience before they become the "less than" that they are judged by others to be?

Often, through the function Ying qi, we recognize the essential need to be part of a whole, so we may create or gather like-minded souls and build a community. If we cannot find acceptance in the society in which we live, then we must build our own society, do what we can to nourish it and help it to grow in the hope that it will become large enough and healthy enough to support the truth of who we are. This requires us to have empathy and compassion for ourselves first and then for those who judge us. We must also have the self-awareness to create exceptionally clear boundaries on what is acceptable in this place. Without boundaries, we will be forced into digesting the judgment of others and then suppressing the feelings associated with that judgment. Forgiving those who judge us is not the same as allowing them to continue to perpetuate their violence upon us. Forgiving is not forgetting. The Ying qi and its association to the Spleen will hold the memory, so we don't forget. The Heart can then help us to let go of the burden of the hate or anger we feel in response to the judgment and find compassion.

Once we are free from the resentment, we have choice. If we are unable to do this, then we may need to create some latency, so that we may survive the overwhelming emotion of it all. The latency created for these types of challenges is created in the Luo-collaterals.

LUO-COLLATERALS

The Luo-collateral system circulates Ying qi and is associated with the distribution of blood and the creation of new blood vessels for the purpose of self-preservation. When our emotions or experiences become too overwhelming to digest or release, we must, at all costs, maintain survival by protecting the organs. So the Luo-collaterals function by creating more blood vessels, usually in the periphery of the body or as far away from the organs as is possible, to protect organ function. By moving blood far away from the organs, they also move the emotions or memories of challenging experiences residing in the blood towards the limbs and surface of the body.

When you internalize an experience, it enters your blood. If the experience is nourishing or if you can learn something useful from it, then the blood continues to circulate and you keep growing. If the experience evokes emotions that are toxic or overwhelming, then we must create distance for self-preservation. The Luo system creates a "holding" vessel.

This creation is visible on the surface of the body in the form of small, superficial vessels, engorged veins or dark discoloration of the skin in the area of the Luo. Look down at the medial aspect of your ankles, in the region of the Kidney Luo point (Ki-4). If you are over the age of 40, it is highly likely that you will find some small superficial vessels that range in color from red to deep purple. These are Luo vessels and they are evidence of your life-long struggle to deal with fear. If you live long enough, at some point you will experience more fear than you can process, and you will need to create some latency. Unprocessed experiences like fear are held in place in the blood until they can be released. This form of latency is designed to hide the uncomfortable experiences away from the conscious mind so that we can continue on until we can gather the resources or perspective needed to manage those experiences in a way that they can be incorporated or released.

This is meant to be a short-term method of holding it all together until we can deal with it. This is very much associated with the Pericardium and the loop of tension that circles the chest, protecting the Heart. Everything you experience in the world that triggers an emotional response is filtered through this band around the chest that protects your Heart. The Pericardium can therefore be very effective for dealing with emotions, until it is overwhelmed by life's experiences. If the Pericardium cannot bear it, you will create latency to survive.

The mental aspect of this process is associated with the Spleen. The Spleen houses the Yi, which is the mental aspect that controls thoughts, ideas and cognition. The Spleen's transformation and transportation function is part of the process of *assimilation* and, with the Yi, it gives *context* to our experiences. The Spleen's strong relationship with the Heart, linked by qi and blood, is what allows the Heart to process emotion in a healthy way. Since the Heart, Pericardium and Spleen have strong associations with blood and therefore Ying qi, their functions are linked to the functions of the Luo-collateral system.

The Luo-collaterals functionally exist in the face of challenges to the body's self-defense systems. They are created and active when we cannot process what is happening to us.

The need for latency can be triggered by an assault from the outside or by an internally generated threat. In the former, it can occur when the Wei qi fails to meet a challenge from the outside. External pathogenic factors are usually dispelled by Wei qi through the Sinew channels. If the Wei qi is too weak or if the pathogen is too strong, then it will move inward and Ying qi will be engaged. This can happen with any of the external pathogenic factors (wind, cold, heat, dry, damp and summer-heat) but it can also occur if we ingest something from the outside (alcohol, tainted food, etc.). The Wei qi will move inward, through the Fu organs and try to rid the body of the pathogen. The nature of Wei qi is yang, so it uses yang qi (heat) to create sweating, peristalsis, urination or defecation, engaging the Fu organs in an attempt to rid the body of the pathogen. Even if the Wei qi is successful, the heat depletes Ying qi. Have you ever had a hangover? The dry mouth and other signs of dehydration such as headache are evidence that the Ying qi has been depleted by the Wei qi attempt to rid us of the toxin. If the Wei qi is not successful or if we override the Wei qi by drinking way too much or doing this too often, then Ying qi, through the Luo system, is engaged to "hold" the pathogen to preserve organ function. A hangover is evidence that our Ying qi and Wei qi did everything they could to save our sorry asses. It is something to be grateful for, even though we may wish we were dead.

You can often see these Luo vessels in people who chronically drink too much. They can be found in many areas of the body but they are especially visible across the nose in an area where many yang channels meet.

The second way that the Luos can be engaged is through the Primary channels. This is typically related to emotional pathogens and lifestyle choices. These internal pathogenic factors initially affect the Primary channels. We know, for instance, that anger injures the Liver and worry injures the Spleen. This is a problem since organ function is important to survival. If the Primary channel cannot resolve or eliminate the emotional distress, it will work to protect the organs and the authenticity of life by creating a holding vessel. The Luo vessel will expand and hold the distraction for as long as the system supplies enough Ying qi and blood for this function.

If the body is weak or if resources are compromised, the Luo will eventually "empty" the pathogen back into the Primary channels. This means we can hold on to a toxic emotional experience for a long time or, at the very least, until we lack the resources to maintain the hold or until our resources are needed elsewhere to deal with a more serious threat.

There are 16 Luo vessels. That is significantly more than the other systems. I like to imagine that the Architect of Humanity somehow understood the need for an abundance of vessels in this system to help us deal with the onslaught of experience.

The Luo-collaterals have three aspects: Longitudinal, Transverse and Deep. For the sake of our conversation on self-preservation, we are most interested in the Longitudinal Luos. That does not mean that the others play no part in survival; they do. The Deep Luos connect to the organs through the Transverse Luos. These Luos provide blood to the smaller networking vessels that supply the organs. You can think of them as governing micro-circulation.

The Transverse Luos connect yin and yang paired channels through the Luo and source points. These Luos mediate the relationship between Ying qi and Yuan qi. You might think of the Transverse Luos as shunts that allow for the movement of qi transversely, connecting the Luo point of a channel to the source point of its paired channel. For example, the Lung and Large Intestine channels are connected transversely from the Luo point of the Lungs (Lu-7) to the source point of the Large Intestine (LI-4) and also from Large Intestine Luo (LI-6) to the Lung channel at its source point (Lu-9). In this way, we mediate the relationship between Ying qi and Yuan qi as a way of diverting resources to support function.

The Longitudinal Luos occupy the space between the Primary channels and the surface of the body. In general, with a couple of notable exceptions, they roughly follow the pathways of their associated Primary channels. These vessels mediate the relationship between Ying qi and Wei qi and are therefore of great interest when it comes to internalizing and/or releasing experience. Because of their circulatory and venting functions and because these vessels are capable of supporting latency for self-preservation, they are ideal for supporting patients during times of transition. When we are stuck in latency, treating these vessels can help us to let go of that which no longer serves us. This can help patients let go of their resistance to change.

The downside of this type of latency is that it creates qi and blood stagnation and requires resources to maintain it. You cannot keep something in latency without assigning resources to keep it there. It would be a little like telling your dog to sit, then leaving it in place and assuming it will continue to sit where you left it...all day or forever. Even well-trained dogs cannot resist their nature forever and will eventually move. While you are there paying attention to them, they may try to follow your direction and overcome their nature. But, left unsupervised, they will return to that nature. Qi, whether it is righteous or pathogenic, is by its very nature dynamic. So if you try to trap qi in an area of the body, then you must supply resources (blood and fluids) to keep it there, as by its very nature it wants to move. The struggle of the qi to move from where you have trapped it will cause symptoms that reflect that drive to move. Patients who are suffering from Luo pathology may have some of the following symptoms:

- heat (especially Ying and Xue stage)

- psycho-emotional issues (emotional stagnation/obstruction in process)

- lifestyle issues (suffering arising from self-sabotaging decision-making)

- digestive dysfunction (inability to assimilate life)

- cardiovascular conditions (inability to harmoniously balance circulation)

- pain (qi stagnation, blood stasis, heat or cold)

- lipomas, cysts, tumors, goiter (fluids used to maintain latency)

- bleeding (due to heat, blood stasis or failure to hold)

- increased vascularization (petechiae, spider veins/nevi, varicosities, caput medusa).

The physical symptoms can be found near the Luo point or along the trajectory of the Longitudinal Luo. The emotional symptoms feel like stuckness or resistance to change. It often feels a little as though maintaining the status quo is less risky or threatening than the unknown of letting go. We hold on to our suffering for as long as we can because we are accustomed to this suffering; if we let go, we cannot predict what will happen next. The unknown can be scary.

These symptoms will remain until we are ready to let go of that which we are holding on to or until we run out of resources to maintain it. When we are holding on to this latency, it is called "fullness" in the Luos. When we run out of resources to maintain the latency or if our resources are distracted by something more important, the pathogen or pathogenic experience then "empties" back into the Primary channel system. This is called "emptiness" in the Luo. As the Luos are emptying, the pathogen or that which has been held now moves back into the areas of the body that connect to the organs. In this emptying process, the body still struggles hard to keep this pathogen at bay, so it may make a last-ditch effort to keep the pathogen in place by surrounding it with fluids. This often results in swellings such as nodules, lipomas and goiter.

Issues that relate to the Luo vessels are about the unconscious drive to hold on to that which distracts us from being truly who we are and who we are meant to be. We hold on to these distractions through the blood. We hold on to them because we are unable to face the pain caused by them. When we can release these vessels, by releasing the blood, we may be more capable of manifesting the things in life that allow us to be authentic. We can manifest more authenticity because we, once again, have access to the support of post-natal resources that have been previously used to hold the latency.

The 16 Luo vessels work in three specific areas of influence. There are 12 Luos that influence the 12 Primary channels. There are two Greater Luos associated with the Spleen and Stomach and they influence the chest and hypochondriac region. There are two Constitutional Luos associated with the Ren and Du mai. They influence the 8 EV and the constitution.

Although there are differing opinions in the classical texts about the nature of the flow in these vessels, when it comes to self-preservation, I prefer to think of them as Ying qi vessels that follow the flow of the Ying qi cycle. The first 12 flow as follows: Lung, Large Intestine, Stomach, Spleen, Heart, Small Intestine, Urinary Bladder, Kidney, Pericardium, San Jiao, Gall Bladder and Liver. Most of us learned this flow as the 24-hour meridian clock, starting with the Lungs at 3–5 a.m. and ending with the Liver at 1–3 a.m. The flow begins with the Lungs, the organ system that initiates internalization of experience through the breath, and ends with the Liver channel at Lv-14 in the hypochondrium.

From the region of the diaphragm, we can then see the connection to the Greater Luos of the Spleen (Sp-21) and Stomach (Xu Li). These Greater Luos strongly influence the chest and diaphragm, and they function to keep the pathogen from entering the constitution. They support the Pericardium's ability to constrict the chest to stop movement. I think it is no accident that the two Greater Luos are associated with the organs of digestion. It is as if the system is giving us one last chance to digest or reject an experience before it becomes part of who we are.

From the area around the chest and hypochondrium, the flow moves into the midline and enters the constitution at Ren-15 and then moves downward to Du-1. Once the pathogen has moved into this level, it is more threatening to life because this is the level of Yuan qi and the constitution.

This flow allows us to see how experience is processed. Not all experience that initiates the need to create latency starts on the outside with the Lungs. Some latency is created based on overwhelming emotional experiences that begin on the inside and threaten organ function. Latency can be created anywhere there is overwhelm or vulnerability.

Each of the Luos has specific functions that are basically designed to support or preserve organ function, and pathology in any of them represents the price paid for creating latency. For instance, if the Lungs are overwhelmed by some experience, when the latency is created, it happens along the pathway of the Lung Luo. The pathway begins at Lu-7, passes over the pad of the thumb (Lu-10) and ends in the center of the palm at Pc-8. One of the costs of creating latency in this Luo is increased vascularization in the hands which creates hot palms. One of the common signs of that pathology is small superficial blood vessels found typically on the thumb pad.

The 12 Luos associated with the Primary channels can be grouped into three circuits. These circuits manage three major stages of development (dependency, independence and interdependence). Latency created in any circuit causes a disruption to the development of that stage.

The first circuit includes the first four channels in the Ying qi cycle—the Lung, Large Intestine, Stomach and Spleen. This circuit represents how we struggle with the state of *dependency*. From the moment of birth, we are dependent on others to meet our survival needs. These are the basic needs associated with hunger, comfort and safety. We must learn, before we can even speak, to find a way to communicate our needs, and once communicated, we must find a way to deal with the response to our communication. We alter the nature of our cry to try to get our caregiver to understand what we need. Anyone who has ever cared for an infant can tell you that there are distinctly different cries for pain, hunger and a wet diaper. If our caregiver cannot understand the communication or perhaps even ignores it, then we develop an understanding of the world based on that response. If our caregiver is responsive and caring, then we tend to think of the world as a safe place and we are instinctively satisfied that we have enough or that we are being heard. When the opposite is true, then the world is a stressful place and we feel deprived. This sense of deprivation can linger long into adulthood and may result in a fear-based attitude that reflects the childhood experience. No matter how much we have, it is never enough, which to others may look like greed, but it really comes from a deep-seated belief that develops when our cries are not heard, when our survival needs are not met. These needs are not just related to food and water. They also include comfort items like shelter and warmth. We also need the appropriate balance of sensory stimulation in order to survive. We need touch and we need our senses to be engaged. If we are deprived of these needs, we will suffer enough to create latency. If we receive the needs in a way that is toxic or overwhelming, we will suffer. This does not even need to seem like abuse. We may be raised by two working parents who do not have the ability to give us quality time. We will feel the lack of their presence in our lives, leading to feelings of deprivation. We may have parents who believe they are supporting our growth by keeping us engaged, but in many ways this level of constant activity may disrupt the function of the first circuit. It may overwhelm the nervous system, altering the threshold of response. We may become wired to expect activity, feeling helpless and adrift if we are not busy. We may also just short-circuit from all of the activity and withdraw for the sake of self-preservation. Any of these may result in the need to create latency in the Luos of the first circuit. You may treat all four Luos, and in doing so, you will help the patient deal with the issues around dependency and feelings of deprivation. You may also be able to see that the first circuit issue is related to latency in just one or two of the Luos in this circuit. Each individual Luo plays its part in this process. Understanding the individual functions allows you to narrow your focus on just one.

Functions of the individual Luos
Lu-7
The Lung Luo represents our need to experience. Through the breath, we take in the outside world. Since the lungs disseminate Wei qi to the surface of the body, this is our first contact with the

world around us. Through inhalation, we bring the outside in. Through exhalation, we release that which no longer serves us. The Po/Corporeal Soul governs a reflexive response to the outside world. This reflexive response is driven by the energetics of survival. How much sensation can we experience and still keep going? If we are overwhelmed by sensation at this level, the first thing we do is stop breathing so deeply. If that doesn't work, then we create latency in the Lung Luo. The cost of the latency is an inability to deal with sensation. We may see fidgeting, unusual body sensations or uncomfortable heat sensations in the palms/wrists. The lack of movement that results from creating the latency may cause chest pain or the Lung qi to rebel. The blood that is used to create the latency might try to move, resulting in the coughing of blood. Some patients who have Lung Luo pathology have a constant need for stimulation or interaction with the world. They can never have enough, even if what they are experiencing is too much. They are constantly "grabbing" life; more, more, more.

LI-6

The Large Intestine Luo has a pathway that generally follows the Large Intestine primary pathway. When it arrives in the cheek, it splits into two branches; one branch angles towards the mouth and the other towards the ear. This Luo has a powerful impact on the function of the jaw. It represents our attempts to perceive the world around us. We "chew" over our perceptions and we begin to assimilate the information we are bringing in. With the teeth and jaw, our ability to sense the world is moving inside, internalizing. This is the reason that parents "childproof" their homes. Once a child is on the move, everything it finds will go right into the mouth. Chewing is an early or primitive attempt at learning. When we try to assimilate and increase our knowledge of the world around us, we often bite off more than we can chew. The creation of latency in this Luo taxes the jaw. We see increased biting and chewing often to the point of toothache. These patients are big gum-chewers, or they may constantly have a toothpick in their mouths. They may suffer from bruxism or clenching of the jaw. They might have lesions on the skin inside their cheeks from constantly chewing on that tissue. The increased attempt at assimilation often comes with increased sensitivity. Trying to perceive too much too fast is overwhelming to the senses; so much so that patients may even develop hearing loss. This may be actual diminished hearing or selective hearing loss, where they cannot take in any more.

St-40

The Stomach Luo is the next in this Ying qi flow. In general, this Luo follows the Primary channel until it gets to the face. It passes through the cheek, ascends to the forehead, meets Du-20 and then crosses the midline and descends to St-9. This Luo has the strongest connection to the survival issues in the first circuit. Once we have chewed on everything, we must swallow and move the experience into the stomach. We go beyond the perception of the LI Luo, to having "gut" feelings about the experience. These are feelings that are somewhat instinctual or primitive in nature. They bypass rational or intellectual thought. Sometimes you just know, in your gut, that something is wrong, even if it doesn't make sense. We are beginning to digest the experience. This allows us to discern our feelings about it. We are beginning to label or name an experience in terms of these primitive emotions. This is often why intense childhood experiences or trauma cannot be easily overcome through intellectual investigation, such as talk therapy. When we are traumatized in childhood, our digestive function is still developing, so the imprint of that trauma is strongly emotional and not very amenable to resolution through intellectual processing alone. It would be great to be able to trust our gut, but once we have created latency in this Luo, we are also creating stagnation which makes our gut feelings less trustworthy.

The adrenals are affected in this process. The lack of trust in our instincts may put us in a continual state of "fight or flight."

As a result, we are unable to manage our feelings. We will have difficulty overcoming the feelings with logic. The pathway has a strong influence on the head. When the latency is released, we can begin to think clearly and we are less overwhelmed by emotion. This makes St-40 a very useful point in the treatment of anxiety and panic attacks.

Like the function of the whole first circuit, Stomach Luo pathology is related to a fear of deprivation. That deprivation is directly related to whatever needs we believe are essential to survival. That could be food or shelter, but it also might be love or support that is lacking in sufficient quantity to keep us alive. When we create latency in this Luo, we do it because our emotions are out of control and we cannot find enough comfort to feel safe.

Sp-4

The Spleen Luo follows the Spleen pathway from Sp-4, up the medial aspect of the leg, and when it arrives at the trunk, it moves towards the midline to connect with Ren-12. The Spleen takes the gut feelings of the Stomach and puts them into context. The Yi or spirit of the Spleen provides a matrix of rational thought to support or balance the emotions. It helps us to understand why we do what we do. The Spleen sets the stage for the development of habits. These habits help us to develop intelligence through repetition. When we have an experience, we make associations based on previous events that help us to negotiate our current emotional distress. This process allows us to learn from our experiences. This is possible because the Spleen banks the imagery of the experience by using Ying qi to hold the blood in the vessels. We can learn from what we are able to remember.

The Spleen also aligns our experiences with social agreements. In the effort to fit in and be socially acceptable, we may create context for our experiences based on how others judge our behavior. If someone laughs at you for picking your nose in public, you learn to pick your nose in private so your feelings don't get hurt.

You might also learn to separate your feelings from the judgment of others. Your Spleen helps you to catalog and remember the hurt so that you can learn from it.

When we create latency in this Luo, we have difficulty digesting experience well enough to learn something from it. Context for learning is out of reach. We end up in thought loops that are obsessive in nature. We ruminate to no good end. When we are unable to create enough context to learn and if we cannot learn, it creates distress. The distress then causes us to create latency in this Luo.

When challenging or overwhelming experiences affect the first circuit, we fail to learn what we need to learn about what it means to be dependent on others for survival. This is the "no man is an island" circuit. It is a good thing to be independent, but we must also learn how to ask for help. We need to be able to communicate our needs to others. We also need to learn how to self-soothe when we feel deprived, instead of seeing catastrophe when we don't get what we think we need.

Some people are driven to accumulate vast amounts of money and stuff, and yet no matter how much they have, they are not satisfied. They cannot fill the dark hole of deprivation that drives the urge to accumulate. My mother grew up in Scotland during a time of scant resources. After World War II, rationing was still part of daily life. My mom told us of a time, in her youth, when she had very practical (her word was "ugly") shoes. Because resources were limited, the shoes had to be practical and sturdy so they would last. By the time I was a young adult, my parents had immigrated to the USA and they were doing a bit better financially. My mother discovered Payless Shoes. This discount shoe store turned my mother into a mini version of Imelda Marcos. She accumulated hundreds of pairs of shoes and this need for shoes continued throughout her life.

In my mother's case, this was more related to the Stomach Luo than the other three in this circuit. As is true of Stomach Luo pathology, my mom had some difficulty controlling her emotions.

She was a loving, funny and kind person, but when she was overwhelmed, she would lose it and the air would turn blue. The swearing was how we knew to leave the room, because shortly after the swearing began, she would throw things. To be fair, my mom cannot defend herself, since she is gone now. She was not an angry person and she did not lose her temper often. She did not physically abuse us. In fact, you could say she taught us how to avoid hostile situations. Her life wasn't particularly easy and she handled most of it with acceptance and a sense of humor, but at times that was difficult. My mother loved us in that deep and almost painful way that moms do. I sometimes feel sad that both she and my dad spent so much of their lives trying to overcome the deprivation of their childhoods. It shaped me in a way. I have a different measure of success because of them.

The second circuit of the Luos includes the Heart, Small Intestine, Urinary Bladder and Kidney. This circuit represents our efforts towards *independence*. The relationship between Shao Yin and Tai Yang demonstrates the ability to know oneself and express that knowledge outwardly into the world. This circuit is about "adulting." What does it take to be your own person? This circuit represents the development of the social skills that allow us to live independently and harmoniously with others. Imagine the process a college freshman goes through in their first year at college. They are away from the safety and structure of home, with a roommate who is a virtual stranger. How well they manage that transition is a function of the second circuit. Will they depend on the values they received at home or will they begin to establish their own values that may or may not be in alignment with how they were raised? This circuit requires us to have enough self-awareness that we can individuate and develop autonomy.

Ht-5

This Luo travels from the Luo point up the medial aspect of the arm, influencing the axilla, chest, throat and inner canthus of the eye.

We create latency in the Heart Luo when we are unable to deal with challenges to self-awareness. The Heart supports the awareness of our thoughts and feelings as they are happening. It is constantly striving for transformation and growth, and letting go of that which does not serve that evolution. Along with self-awareness, the Heart has the capacity for unconditional love, empathy and compassion. It supports the ability to clearly communicate thoughts and feelings. Once the latency is created and movement in the chest stops, patients will complain of chest oppression, and pain or fullness in the diaphragm. This constraint is most often associated with feelings of betrayal and the inability to release toxic emotions. Consciousness and communication will be compromised. The Luo point Ht-5 is frequently used for speech problems, especially those related to emotional disruptions of speech, such as stuttering.

SI-7

This Luo follows the SI channel pathway from SI-7 up to the shoulder. The Small Intestine separates pure from turbid, "sorting" things out and trying to get the most value out of them. Its job is to absorb what is nutritious and reject waste. The Small Intestine is using discernment to create clarity. It integrates information and provides feedback to the Heart, giving the Heart another opportunity for awareness. When we create latency in this Luo, it is because our sorting function has gone wrong. Our ability to discern what is useful is impaired. This lack of discernment creates chaos and a sense of order is lost. The cost of that latency is a need to control our world through over-sorting. If we could just get this sorted out, then peace and order will be restored. Unfortunately, order on the outside does not ensure order on the inside. On the other hand, the drive to sort might be useful if we want to clean and organize our closets. The failure to re-establish order from the chaos can make us rigid, critical and overbearing. We are driven to control others, so their chaos doesn't amplify ours. One would be wise to avoid disrupting the artificial sense of order created by someone with Small Intestine Luo pathology. Never move things on their desk or return things to the wrong place. This external order is creating the illusion of internal order; disrupting that destroys the illusion and the sense of peace. I am reminded of a time in my life, many years ago, when my Small Intestine was overwhelmed. I was newly married and living with two teenage boys and I had a hard time adjusting. I became very critical of their lifestyle and the perceived disruption to mine. It became so challenging for me that I bought a label-maker and labeled my kitchen cupboards and drawers. I would have order. Not that it helped, but I can look back on that now and see how badly I handled that adjustment and how I created latency in the Small Intestine that resulted in a constant need for approval, mostly from myself, and an inability to find a way out of the chaos. It was challenging for us all.

UB-58

This Luo descends from UB-58 to connect with the Kidney channel at Ki-3, where it follows the path of the Kidney Luo ending at the diaphragm. The Urinary Bladder (Foot Tai Yang) is the largest Yang channel that engages the exterior. Think of it as an early warning system that sets the threshold of response to external stimuli. The Bladder channel has a lot of influence on what information gets in. This allows us to see only what we want to see, so it impacts the integrity of our experiences. If, for instance, you hear a loud bang, such as a door slamming or car engine backfiring, it is a normal response to reflexively turn or even move towards the place where the noise came from. This is the Tai Yang/Wei qi way of saying, "What just happened?" If you are living in a state of fear or anxiety, it is more likely that instead of moving towards the noise, you will duck or run. In this fearful state, the Bladder channel anticipates danger and the survival instinct kicks in. There is no curiosity about what has just happened; there is only a reaction meant to preserve life. The assumption is made that the noise indicates a threat because, in a state of anxiety, threat is everywhere.

If, on the other hand, you have lived in an area where loud noises are commonplace, such as a war zone or a neighborhood where major road construction or new building is happening, the Bladder channel will do its best to use qi and fluids to buffer the input of the sound, and you might not even hear it after a while. There is a range of responses to external stimuli and the Bladder channel is supposed to set the appropriate response to that input. If it decides that the input is overwhelming, then it will work to block the input to help us maintain sanity. The need to create latency may result in hypervigilance, panic attacks or hyperventilation. The cost of creating latency in this Luo is congestion that blocks both perception and response. If the threat is great or ongoing, the fluid congestion, which typically starts in the head, will eventually spread body-wide. This is obesity or systemic edema that acts as a buffer against perceived threat.

Ki-4

The Kidney is injured by fear. How much can we take and still have the will to live? This fear is that deep survival-based fear that causes symptoms such as PTSD, panic attacks, phobias or any fear that makes us feel as if we could die. The fear negatively affects our ability to trust. The pathway of this Luo rises from the medial aspect of the ankle at the Luo point (Ki-4) to the diaphragm connecting to the Pericardium loop. Pathology in the Kidney Luo affects this Kidney–Pericardium relationship and makes it difficult to trust that being in the world is safe. Without the trust, each time the fear is experienced, it is like the first time. When you release this Luo, it is very common to see people take a deep cleansing breath and relax.

The struggle to become your own person is a second-circuit issue. You might see this in a patient who is still living at home, long after the age of independence. I know that in many places in the world generations of families all live in the same house. I am not talking about that. I am saying that the need to stay home or be dependent on our parents may be limiting our ability to be fully autonomous individuals.

I also see patients stuck in latency involving the second-circuit struggle with what might be known as "prosperity consciousness." They are independent but somehow they are unable to find their worth. They seem to be able to manage the resources for survival (first circuit) but they do not feel worthy of abundance.

The remaining circuit is composed of the Pericardium, San Jiao (Triple Warmer), Gall Bladder and Liver. The first circuit represents the struggle with dependency, the second with independence and the third circuit represents a struggle with *inter-dependence*. In the second circuit, the struggle for independence requires a level of self-awareness or self-knowing. In the third circuit, the issue is self-differentiation. I know who I am but how does that fit in with everyone else? How will I deal with the expectations and value judgments of others? What can I offer to my community? What unique characteristics do I bring that can define my usefulness? This circuit reflects our ability to manage the stress and emotions that are triggered by our interactions with others. The self-preservation here is less immediately about physical survival and more about emotional survival and the ability to maintain our sense of self while facing the judgments and expectations of others.

Pc-6

This Luo ascends the arm from Pc-6, crosses the chest to the midline and then descends through all three jiaos. The Pericardium, as the Heart protector, is responsible for the mediation of thoughts, feelings and actions that are meant to preserve the sovereignty of the Emperor. It is about the capacity for self-preservation and the development of a coping style that helps us to negotiate challenging social interaction. When it is functioning well, we have an appropriate response to criticism. We can maintain intellectual control over our emotions and through this we can develop self-esteem. We don't take criticism personally. When we are being criticized, the Pericardium gives us the capacity to find the useful feedback in the criticism and let the rest go, knowing it has nothing to do with us. The Pericardium creates a language for processing our emotions and it helps us to maintain our sanity through rationalization. It helps us to redirect our emotions for self-preservation. If we are hurt or disappointed by an interaction, then the Pericardium will help us to rationalize the experience so that we can let it go. Latency is created when we can no longer rationalize the hurt. The stagnation that occurs in the creation of latency constricts the Pericardium loop, causing chest pain or restriction of breathing. The ability to process the emotions that are triggered by interaction with others is impaired. When we cannot process our emotional experiences, we may become disconnected from our emotions. It is not uncommon to then look outside ourselves at the emotional experiences of others. This may make us feel overprotective or overly concerned with the emotional status of the people around us, even though we cannot control or alter their experience. In a sense, this is a distraction that helps us to avoid the suffering we feel at being disconnected from our own emotions. The cost of this latency is a defensiveness that leads to despair. When we cannot rationalize the emotional experience of ourselves or others, we may feel attacked, as if the whole world is against us.

SJ-5

This Luo pathway rises from SJ-5, up the arm, across the shoulder into the chest and down through all three jiaos. The San Jiao is the avenue of Yuan qi and the official in charge of irrigation. This channel has a strong connection through Yuan qi to our constitution or temperament. Latency is created in this channel when there are challenges to who we are or how we are in the world. Although the San Jiao disseminates Yuan qi to all three jiaos, the yin–yang connection to the Pericardium increases its ability to influence the upper jiao, especially the lungs. This upper jiao connection is supposed to facilitate release. When latency is created, the chest tightens and that release is impeded. As we get closer to the constitution, the pathogenic experiences become deeper and more easily confused with Self. That makes them more challenging to release. We might be stubborn in our resistance to letting go. The confusion with Self also makes us more rigid in our stance and less relatable to others. Decision-making becomes more difficult. Conditions that develop because of the latency are very close to entering the constitution, so they are more difficult to resolve. We see intractable diseases at this level of latency. Many cancers begin at this level. Many cancers begin at this level with cell mutation that might be considered a perversion of Yuan qi. This alteration of Self happens when stress and lifestyle choices force the creation of latency in the San Jiao.

GB-37

This is the second Luo that moves distally away from the trunk. The pathway moves from GB-37, down the leg, across the foot to St-42. The other Luo that moves distally is the Lung Luo. They share a quality of release. The Gall Bladder gives us the courage needed to release. The Shao Yang nature of the Gall Bladder gives us the ability to turn our heads and open our peripheral vision. This allows us to see more options and new possibilities or maybe just to see something in a totally different light. The Gall Bladder is a Curious Organ and, as such, it has a link to the 8 EV. Once again, we are talking about pathogens getting closer to the constitution. The need to release is becoming a little more urgent and desperate. Latency is created when our courage fails us and we feel defeated. We may feel victimized or find it easier to blame others for the situation we are in. We might also feel so overcome that our legs are too weak to hold our weight; rising from a sitting position may even stress us to the point of fainting. There is despair and a sense of hopelessness that makes us want to withdraw from the world. As we lose the flexibility of the Gall Bladder that comes from the nature of Wood, we see people stuck in a perception of self that is narrow and sort of "all or nothing." We cannot even imagine another way to be. The frustration that comes with this will make change more challenging.

Lv-5

The Liver Luo ascends the medial aspect of the leg from Lv-5 and terminates in the region of the genitals. This is the last Luo in the Ying qi cycle. The Liver governs the capacity for judgment. We need this capacity to know where we stand and how to engage the world around us. This is a little like playing Poker. We are dealt a hand. We have to determine how to play that hand but we must also assess or "judge" the intent of the other players. Sometimes you just need to "fold" your hand and walk away and sometimes you need to "go all in." This is a Liver function. This is a Liver function. Latency is created when the world is judged as a hostile place. There is no sense of peace and we are filled with uncertainty. The stagnation that results from this latency often obstructs the lower jiao, causing fullness in the genital region. Sexual arousal is no longer about intimacy or love; it is linked to frustration, anger and resentment. Even though we might want intimacy and connection, we are too angry to be vulnerable enough to allow the intimacy to happen. We connect in angry ways.

The third circuit reflects our ability to negotiate the emotional challenges of relationship. You might see this in a person who has great success in all the measures of independence. They may be financially secure, own their own home or business, but they have a string of failed relationships. They struggle with intimacy. They are perhaps too independent and cannot negotiate the fears and risks of inter-dependence. You might also see this in someone who is very skilled but they cannot hold on to a job because they have difficulty getting along in the workplace.

At this point, the movement of the pathogen has completed the Ying qi cycle and should move into the constitution at Ren-15.

We have one last opportunity to prevent that and try to release it. That opportunity comes through the Greater Luos of the Spleen and Stomach (Sp-21 and Xu Li). These two Luos affect the movement in the chest through the Pericardium loop. If we can support the circulation in the chest and diaphragm, then maybe we can release that which we are holding on to. This is a sort of last-ditch attempt to release something that will pervert our Yuan qi if it manages to enter our constitution through the Ren and Du. This is about having an experience so injurious or so overwhelming that it bypasses all of the earlier attempts at release and becomes embodied as Self. If we can't let it go through the Greater Luos, it will become part of who we are.

Sp-21

The Greater Luo of the Spleen may be considered the gateway to the constitution. The pathway spreads out across the flank and chest from Sp-21. Once latency is created here, existence becomes painful. As we are knocking on the door to the constitution, we become more and more depressed, and we begin to lose hope that the situation we find ourselves in might ever be resolved. There is often widespread somatization of emotional pain. Everything hurts, but there is often little wrong with the actual physical structure and function of the body. These people have heard, many times, "There is nothing wrong with you." They have heard it so often that they begin to feel as if they are going crazy. It takes a very long time to get a diagnosis. They may be given psychiatric drugs to manage their pain because opiates are typically ineffective for this type of pain. This type of latency and the pain it causes may be seen in patients diagnosed with fibromyalgia. They feel beaten down, victimized and quite often as if they are being martyred—that their suffering is not just about them anymore. Eventually, this pain is so consuming that patients turn on themselves and suffer from self-loathing and thoughts of self-harm. Part of the problem with something like fibromyalgia or chronic fatigue is that there is no visible sign of the excruciating pain. Patients may eventually be driven to thoughts of creating wounds that are visible to all. Eventually, the inability to maintain the latency may result in suicidal ideation. These patients are losing the will to live.

Xu Li

The Greater Luo of the Stomach is the only unilateral point in the Primary channel system. It can be found only on the left side of the body over the apex of the Heart. The apical heartbeat can be felt under this point. Because it is located in the tissue of the breast, it is not needled in practice. Latency in this Luo may be addressed in the area near the point. Lv-14 or St-18 can be useful to this end or you can look for the small superficial vessels on the skin in the region. If there are no obvious vessels, we will usually treat this Luo through the 8 EV. The typical choice for this is the Chong or Yin Wei because of their influence on the chest.

This Luo vessel has a pathway that connects the Stomach to the diaphragm and Heart. The most common symptoms of latency in this Luo are anxiety and palpitations. Once the Heart is affected, the ability to be conscious of your emotions is compromised. Pathology trapped in this Luo challenges our ability to assimilate experience in a way that supports the Heart. Feelings of anxiety make it difficult to determine the veracity of threat. We may not be able to tell what is triggering the anxiety. Patients who tell you they have anxiety may not be able to tell you why or where they experience the effect of the anxiety in their bodies.

We have 14 opportunities to deal with overwhelming experiences through post-natal function, from the Lungs through the Greater Luos of the Spleen and Stomach. If we fail to manage it through these vessels, then the pathogen will move into the constitution. The flow moves from the diaphragm towards the midline to Ren-15, the Luo point of the Ren mai. The Ren mai is a jing vessel and it is a reservoir for the primary Yin resources that are pre-natal in nature. Pre-natal jing is the basis for our constitution.

Once this process moves into the constitution, it becomes much more challenging to treat. These Constitutional Luos are about the accumulation of Karma. Unresolved emotional or pathogenic experiences are dumped into jing for processing in the next life or they are passed down to the next generation. It is a way of saying, "I have tried everything I can to let this go and now I am just done with it and I accept that I will die with the weight of this in my bones." Once the pathogen is accepted into this level, it is difficult to distinguish it from Self. Treating the Luo itself may not be enough. You will likely need to regulate, release and restore the function of the 8 EV as well.

Ren-15

The Luo of the Ren mai spreads out across the diaphragm like the tail of a turtledove. From just below the xiphoid process, the function of this Luo is to spread resources across the abdomen. When the Ren mai is healthy, we have access to the yin resources that help us to feel nourished and connected. Ren-15 is the upper point on the Bao Mai (Uterine vessel) which connects the Heart to the Kidneys and the Pericardium loop to the Dai mai. These connections help us to feel embodied enough to make self-care a priority. When there is latency in this Luo, we lose contact with ourselves and we are unable to connect with emotions and sensation through the middle of the trunk. We lose the ability to connect with the stability in the center of the body. This disrupts the connection between the Shen and the Zhi. We have now lost our way because we cannot maintain the sovereignty of the Heart and Kidney axis.

Du-1

From this point, the flow follows the path of the Bao Mai and descends to Du-1, the Luo point of the Du mai. The Du mai is the Sea of Yang which governs all yang functions. Through its influence on the spine, it supports our exploration of the world. Latency in this Luo impacts healthy individuation. It obstructs the ability to take the emotions associated with the Ren and put them into action in a way that expresses a healthy sense of potency and identity. Latency created in this Luo makes it difficult to hold the weight of our heads on our shoulders. We lose the potency of yang for locomotion and exploration. We will find it difficult to maintain an upright posture. We begin to collapse with the weight of our accumulated experience, stored in the brain.

TREATING THE LUOS

The easiest way to see the need for a Luo treatment is through the visible signs of latency. Look for evidence of an increase in superficial blood vessels. These vessels can be found near the Luo point or anywhere along the general flow of the Longitudinal Luo. Sometimes the Luos are congested a little more deeply, under the skin, and therefore the superficial vessels are less distinct. In some patients, the Luos may look like small petechiae or a slight discoloration of the skin in the region of the Luo. This may be a little more difficult to recognize, so there are other reasons to choose a Luo treatment. You can also see evidence of Luo pathology in the way patients process emotional experiences. You can use Luo treatments in patients who are holding on to specific emotions and, even with effort and intention, they cannot let go. For instance, a patient may be aware that the anger they feel is destructive. They may want to let it go, but they find themselves unable to do that. They may tell you they have tried everything. Even if there are no obvious visible vessels near any of the Luos that might deal with this anger, you can still release the Luos.

Luo vessel treatments are also useful in patients struggling with "relationship" issues. Since the Luos are Ying qi vessels, they have influence on how we interact with others. There are also ways to address the three circuits of the Luos if you can see a patient stuck in a stage of development. If, for instance, you have a patient who is struggling with survival issues and they are living in a state of fear based on deprivation, then you can release the Luos in the first circuit.

When we decide to treat the Luos, the most important goal of the treatment is to bring the blood that is stuck in the process of latency up to the surface so the pathogen can be released. The most efficient and immediate way to do that is through bleeding the small superficial vessels. This may be done with a lancet or three-edged needle. I find the lancet a little less aggressive as it makes a smaller hole than the three-edged needle. The bleeding is done whether there is "fullness" or "emptiness" in the Luo. Once latency is created, bringing blood to the surface is the most effective part of treatment. If you or your patient are uncomfortable with bleeding, then you can bring the blood to the surface of the body in other ways. You can use gua sha, plum-blossom needle or cupping. These techniques draw the blood to the surface of the body, making it easier to let go.

If you have determined that the patient has insufficient resources to maintain the latency and the pathogen is "emptying" back into the Primary channel, then you may need to support Yuan qi and organ function. You can do this by adding a source point. This will support organ function and engage the will. You may also use moxa because its warming function supports Yuan qi.

In terms of self-preservation, the true value of the Luo mai is their "network" nature. They allow us to reach into those areas where we have hidden away those experiences or emotions that we think we cannot bear. Using the Luo mai, we can release that which no longer resonates with our authentic selves. Once we free these vessels of the burden of latency, then we will once again have access to the resources that support us in having a life of meaning and purpose. If the motto of the Sinews is "free the body, free the mind," then the motto of the Luos is "free the blood, reclaim your resources."

KEYS TO SELF-HELP FOR YING QI AND THE LUO-COLLATERALS

Breathe

Breath is life, so breathing is an excellent way to self-treat. It is free, effective and does not require any equipment. For Ying qi and the Luo-collaterals, breathing becomes about letting go of emotional stuckness. Breathe in as comfortably deep as you can, and when you exhale, make some noise. Any noise—a hum, a moan, a groan, a yell or a scream. When you make a noise on the exhale, you cause a vibration in the diaphragm and throat that helps facilitate the venting of stuck emotion. When you exhale like this, you support letting go. If you have ever done Laughing Qi Gong, the effect is very similar.

Feel your feelings

The more you try to avoid what you are feeling, the bigger it becomes and the more it persists. Feel them but remember they are an experience you are having. They are not who you are. Find ways to express your emotions creatively: art, journal-writing or creating a garden. Listening to music or playing an instrument can put you in touch with your feelings and give you an outlet for emotions. Watch a sad or poignant movie. *Steel Magnolias* or *The Shawshank Redemption* should do the job nicely.

Increase your circulation

Move your body, circulate your blood. Cardiovascular exercise is helpful here. Get your heart rate up. I am a big fan of dancing it out!

A LUO-COLLATERAL CASE STUDY

The patient is a male in his late 60s. When I first saw this patient, he had been referred to me based on a life-long history of trauma.

On his first visit, he told me he had a dream that it was time for him to work on his mom issues. He had a very challenging relationship with his mom in childhood that he believed led to deep feelings of unworthiness, sadness, anxiety, a string of failed relationships and a long history of drug and alcohol abuse. He had been in recovery for quite some time and felt as if it was time to let go of the trauma. His physical symptoms included nightmares, night sweats, difficulty falling asleep, chronic cough, itching rashes, depression, sinus congestion with allergies, and a significant number of digestive problems related to both Stomach and Spleen deficiencies. He also had a few Kidney symptoms including intermittent tinnitus, hair loss, low back pain and being easily frightened. His pulse was a diaphragm pulse on the left. This pulse has its major force between the first and second fingers. The blockage is felt between the pulses that represent the upper and middle jiao. On the right, his pulse was thready, in the second level and long, felt beyond the third finger. This long straight pulse found in the second level is, according to my pulse teacher Will Morris, consistent with Ren mai pathology. This is not surprising considering my patient's chief complaints were directly related to his relationship to source yin (his mother). His tongue was slightly wide, dusky, and the coat from the midpoint to the root was turbid. I determined that since he wanted to work on the mom issues, the first place to start was a Po treatment for trauma in the first cycle of jing. This treatment begins with the Luo point of the Ren mai (Ren-15) and it is followed by Ren-13, which accesses the first cycle of jing, the age in which the trauma began. I then made a figure 8 or "infinity loop" of Lu-7 and Ki-6, beginning with Lu-7 on the left (the side of pre-natal yin), Ki-6 on the right, Ki-6 on the left and finally Lu-7 on the right. The intent was to release the imprint of the early trauma and start to begin to build a relationship with his own yin. This treatment, as simple as it was, stirred up a rather emotional response, with increased agitation and anxiety.

About five weeks later, he came for his next treatment because he felt that the first treatment gave him much to work through. He had been having a few treatments at one of the local school clinics in which they focused on his digestion and skin rashes. It was determined that he was pre-diabetic. The combined treatments may have overwhelmed his digestion which was already on the weak side. There was increased evidence of heat in both his tongue and his pulse. Since he was having treatments at the school clinic, I decided to continue the 8 EV since this was unlikely to be done in a school clinic and his early trauma had definitely altered his curriculum. He was very determined to improve his awareness. Consciousness was important to him.

The second treatment was a Chong mai treatment to link the pre- and post-natal qi to support digestion. The hope was the Chong mai would help him digest the information being provided in treatments and remind him who he was. The points were: Sp-4, Pc-6, St-36, Ren-7, Ki-21 and Ki-26.

Sp-4: Master point of Chong mai.

Pc-6: Couple point of Chong, master point of Yin Wei.

St-36: He-sea point to support digestion.

Ren-7: Crossing point of Ren and Chong to provide continuity with the first treatment.

Ki-21: For abdominal fullness. Dark Gate is the last point on the darkness of yin in the abdomen before it rises on to the chest. It is also the exit point of the Kidney channel. It clears heat from the Heart and resolves fear of the unknown.

Ki-26: Front-shu of Metal, supports the function of the Po for feelings of agitation and anxiety.

I did not see this patient after that for several months. When he returned, it was because he was experiencing anxiety as a result of a broken friendship. The friendship ended with an episode where he felt verbally attacked by this person that he perceived to be a very close friend. This verbal attack happened in a public setting. He was having a very hard time letting go of the anger and, as a result of that, the skin rashes were worse and he had developed a red and painful stye on his right eye. The rash had spread to the shins, anterior and medial thigh and groin region, and was also spreading over the lateral aspect of the Pericardium loop along the Gall Bladder channel. The Luo treatment that followed was:

Bleed Lv-5 and GB-37.

Needle Ren-7 and Ren-15, right Lv-14, left Lu2 threaded to Lu-1, Du-24.

As a way of maintaining consistency with the original goal of working on mom issues, Ren-7 (crossing point of Chong and Ren) was used to connect the fluids of the Ren with the blood of the Chong.

The combination of Lv-14 with Lu-1 supports starting over. Using the last point on the Liver channel with the first point of the Lung channel says, "Let's begin again."

Du-24, Spirit Courtyard, was added to calm the Shen and open the consciousness.

The patient was then able to see the connection between this relationship and earlier abusive relationships, and the anger was eased and appropriate grief took its place.

The patient had a number of other treatments to continue working on the mom stuff but he did have one more noticeable Luo treatment. Eventually, in the course of his internal exploration, he recognized that he was quite terrified in childhood and that fear became a life-long companion. He had observable vessels, both red and purple, around Ki-4, the Luo point of the Kidney channel. The Kidney Luo rises up from Ki-4 along the medial aspect of the leg and ends at the level of the diaphragm at Ren-15. Just above Ren-15 and spread across the lower ribs, you could easily see a number of Luo vessels. When those vessels were bled, the patient reflexively took a deep cleansing breath and he became deeply relaxed.

This particular patient has a lot of therapeutic tools that are useful for processing the latency as it is released. He was not afraid to experience emotions and use them to learn more about himself. He had a good support system and a therapeutic container that allowed for safer exploration. This was important because, as you will see later in the book, this patient had created a tremendous amount of latency to survive.

WHY CHOOSE A LUO TREATMENT?

As the Sinew channels govern the exterior of the body through the circulation of Wei qi, the Luos govern the interior of the body through the circulation of Ying qi and blood. Deciding to do a Luo treatment means that you have seen changes in the superficial circulation. You have a visible representation of increased vascularization, in the form of small superficial blood vessels on or near the Luo point or somewhere along its path. The acts of self-preservation that create latency for survival in this system may also be associated with any of the following:

- emotional stagnation (especially if one is stuck on a particular emotion)

- difficulty interacting with others

- a broken heart that isn't healing

- difficulty growing in relationship (growth is much easier when no one is pushing your buttons)

- difficulty internalizing life (most often seen in the form of anxiety or depression).

Choosing to do a Luo treatment means that you have decided to give the patient what they need to let go. Bleeding the Luos is a way of releasing that which has become a distraction to living a full and authentic life. It is so easy to say, "Just let it go," but that is like telling someone who is tense everywhere to "just relax." It isn't going to happen. Once we have created this stagnation in the blood, we are resistant to let it go because we are afraid that we will be overwhelmed once again by the emotional experience. We fear that if we let it loose, it will never end. Bleeding the Luos is a way to take the charge out of the emotion by releasing the blood that is holding it.

—— CHAPTER 7 ——

THE PRIMARY CHANNELS

Although it does not have a direct mechanism for creating latency, the Primary channel system plays a very important role in self-preservation. It does this through digestive function. Like the Luo-collateral system, the Primary channels are Ying qi vessels. One of the jobs of nutritive qi (Ying qi) is to make sure we are nourished enough to maintain organ function. Processing life productively and maintaining sufficient resources for sustaining life requires good digestive function. If that digestive function is productive, then we are much less likely to drain our pre-natal resources. In this way, you could say that productive digestion and the resulting healthy organ function support the pursuit of our destiny by preserving the pre-natal resources that are called upon when digestion and organ function fail.

Li Dong Yuan was the founder of the Nourishing Earth School (Spleen and Stomach School). This school was one of the four important medical schools of the Jin and Yuan dynasties. Li Dong Yuan emphasized that the protection of digestive function is the most important principle for prolonging life. When preventing and treating diseases, protection of the Spleen and Stomach should be taken into consideration. Protecting our digestive function is the Primary channel approach to self-preservation. This is accomplished by the regulation of diet, lifestyle and emotions. When we are challenged by life, altering our diet to support digestive function can help us to generate the resources we need to manage the challenge. We also need to find ways to make lifestyle choices that help us to manage stress. Adequate exercise, restorative sleep and a balance between work and play can help us to better assimilate life in a way that supports growth. The decisions we make that elevate our self-care and help us to build a good support system can help us to thrive.

The Earth element is the center of the wheel and it provides a pivot around which all the other elements can transform. Our potential in life is actualized by the Earth's ability to use all available resources needed for nourishment that will support our constitution and temperament. The Earth element helps us to develop healthy boundaries in relation to nourishing our self and others. This is something we typically learn how to do through our relationship with our mothers or primary caregivers. How we are nourished by those who love us has a tremendous impact on our capacity to nourish ourselves and those around us. This relationship has the potential to teach us not only how to nourish ourselves but also how to bond appropriately and create healthy boundaries. If we are fortunate enough to have caregivers who love us and are invested in our growth, then we will likely struggle less with issues related to nourishment. If we are neglected or fed in a way that does not support good health, then our relationship to food is less balanced. If we have mothers who set good boundaries and allow us to individuate when the time comes, then we will grow into adults who have the capacity to set our own boundaries. If we are over-bonded or abandoned, then creating healthy boundaries might be challenging.

The Earth element helps us to develop the capacity for grounding and centering. This is the ability to maintain stability in the face of constant change, challenge and chaos. The spirit of the Spleen engenders stability and the capacity for stillness. Stillness helps us feel our center. Stillness makes us more aware of how grounded we might be in the moment. Before right-action is a moment of stopping. A chance to take a breath and choose.

If we cannot digest well enough to stay grounded and stable, then we will generate dampness to hold the center any way we can. Accumulation of dampness, produced by the Spleen, is an example of over-centering as an attempt to maintain stability. Although this is not the creation of latency, it is an attempt at maintaining enough stability for function to continue. Stubborn weight gain may in some instances be an act of self-preservation.

The Yi (spirit of the Spleen) helps us to focus our attention and intention on those things we need to change so that we may learn and grow. As I mentioned earlier, change is difficult. Once we become habituated in our thoughts and behaviors, it is challenging to learn, grow and change. We can very easily become unconsciously stuck in the safety of the known. It's a little like the movie *Groundhog Day*. Even though we are not having a good time living the same day over and over, we know what is coming next and that feels safer than the risks of the unknown.

Healthy movement is initiated from the middle. Movement that begins in other places is less focused, less stable and less clear in intent. It may be easy to think of change as an idea, but if change is to last, it must become a somatic, embodied experience. We must internalize the change and embrace a new relationship to it. When we get "stuck" in the process of change, we are served by returning to the center. Being centered gives us the capacity to be present to the moment, allowing for an openness and willingness to proceed. Being centered allows us to see what is, so that we can then begin to create an environment through our attention and intention, in which lasting change can occur. All of this happens with the functions governed by the Spleen and Stomach. The center presents an anchoring point around which we can examine what we are sensing and feeling without being carried away by rumination and emotions that have no context for learning.

It is essential to experience the energy from the center down into the legs and the earth. The capacity to ground enhances stability in the face of change. When faced with the need for change, the impulse to move is tainted by the increased risk associated with that change. The body may "freeze," becoming stuck so that change cannot occur, or we may run from the change, moving chaotically and ineffectively. The emotional experience occurring during this time is also chaotic. By moving the energy downward into the legs, we can use the qi of the Spleen and Stomach to come to a place of being present to what is. In this way, we can begin to consciously override the Wei qi response to change and choose actions that will support the change.

The Primary channels are the bread and butter of the acupuncturist's practice. We are all trained how to use this channel system for a wide variety of conditions. There is little I can add in terms of how best to use it for self-preservation. I might, however, suggest that when using this system to address issues of self-preservation, one might consider adding into any treatment points that we know will facilitate digestion. Points that support digestive function also support the ability to digest life. These points and any points that support the Earth element will also enhance stability and grounding. It is hard to beat the primary triangle of the Earth School for this function. Ren-12 is the front-mu point of the Stomach and St-36 is the He-sea point and an Earth point. This triangle is very effective at facilitating a return to the center.

Once the grounding is in place, you might think about points that restore proper directional flow by regulating the qi mechanism. When someone creates dampness as a way of pathologically centering, that dampness will obstruct the appropriate flow of qi. Once the qi flow is obstructed, then change or growth is also blocked. Points on the Ren mai have a very powerful impact on the directional flow of qi, especially Ren-17, Ren-12 and Ren-6. I also like Sp-8, the xi-cleft point of the Spleen channel. This point can restore ascending and descending out of the middle by unblocking stagnation and waking the Spleen.

Consider how to regulate what we take in and how we let go, using points that harmonize Ying and Wei. After stabilizing the middle, regulation of function in the upper jiao (taking in) and the lower jiao (letting go) will help to rectify how patients manage life. It is a reminder that digesting life is easier if we can manage input and facilitate elimination. The points I use most often for this function are Lu-2 threaded to Lu-1 and St-25.

Finally, you might think about how to support organ function by adding points that have a connection to Yuan qi. When we access Yuan qi, we bring constitutional resources to support Ying qi and digestive function. This might include source points, front-mu points, back-shu points and the Kidney-shu points on the chest. Another point combination that I employ for this is SJ-4 and St-42. These are the Yuan-source points of the San Jiao and Stomach. The San Jiao is the avenue of Yuan qi and the official in charge of irrigation. This point facilitates the distribution of Yuan qi for function and the appropriate circulation of fluids. The source point of the Stomach (St-42) strengthens the descending function of the Stomach and regulates digestion. The combination of these two points links together the pre- and post-natal function of the San Jiao and Stomach, creating effective support for digestion. These two points used with the primary triangle of the Earth School (Ren-12 and St-36) seem to be very useful in patients suffering from chronic fatigue.

Undoubtedly, these are points that you are already using with confidence. If what you are doing every day isn't producing the results you had hoped for, or if it works for a while and then progress stalls, having an understanding of these other channel systems can be useful. If you can recognize that latency has been created, then you will see why the Primary channels are not functioning optimally. If you can further discover at which level of qi this latency has been created, then you will know which of the channel systems may be used to free the latency and support the function of the system that nourishes the organs and digests life.

Releasing the latent pathogen frees up resources that are used to support the function of the Primary channels.

As for what you can do to support your own capacity to digest life, the list is endless but you can begin with the following:

- Add more food into your diet that is nutrient-dense. If you have access to locally grown, organic products and you can afford them, even better. Eat the rainbow. Variety in color, taste and texture matters. If you are able, grow your own food and grow it with love and the intent that it will nourish whoever eats it.

- Eliminate things from your diet that you cannot pronounce or that you know irritate your digestion.

- Eat routinely. The Spleen likes repetition and routine. Predictable dietary habits create a sense of stability for the Spleen.

- The Spleen doesn't like cold, so minimize or eliminate cold, raw foods from your diet until your digestion is strong enough to deal with them. I understand that raw foods have more nutrients than cooked ones, but that is only useful if you are able to digest them enough to absorb those nutrients.

- Try to be calmer and more mindful when you eat, and chew more. Digestion begins in the mouth.

- Don't eat too late at night. As yang declines, so does digestive function.

- Remember you are eating for more than your body, so find pleasure in what you ingest.

- Examine what you are taking in and digesting that isn't food. If your input is overwhelming your capacity to digest, then consider reducing it. Watch less news, or scroll Facebook,

Twitter and Instagram less often. Please do not watch these things while you eat.

- Do what you need to do to get enough good-quality sleep. If you are not a great sleeper, then get treatment for that or resign yourself to getting enough rest. You need downtime.

- Meditate or, if you find that difficult, find an activity that you enjoy, such as gardening, and do it mindfully. You can make any activity a meditation.

- Walk barefoot on natural surfaces daily and, when you can, get out into nature.

- Breathe. You know you want to. Set an alarm on your watch or phone twice a day. When it goes off, stop whatever you are doing and take three deep breaths. If you are stressed out, make sure the exhale is longer than the inhale.

- Exercise regularly. First, because it is good for you, but also circulation is important for digestion. Change cannot happen without movement. Walking is a good start.

If you are in survival mode, as many of us are, then right about now, or perhaps even halfway into that list, your Wei qi is screaming, "RED ALERT. The sky is falling, the sky is falling! Run, run, run!" Asking someone to change these things so that they can digest life better triggers the resistance to change that is part of the reptile brain's way of keeping us safe. It is impossible to negotiate the risk that occurs when you ask someone to alter so many things in their life. Pick one or, if you are brave and confident, pick two. Focus on small changes first; then, as those changes become more routine, you can add new changes.

A word about failure. Failure is part of the process of change. When we set an intent to change something and then we move towards that change, sometimes we have bad days where sustaining the change fails. Beating ourselves up for that failure is counterproductive. Change is initiated by setting an intent. This is like flipping a switch. We just decide we are going to do something and then we do it. But change is not sustained in this manner. Change is a process in which we decide each day or each moment to commit to that change until we have done it long enough to make it a routine. This means that some days making the decision to sustain the change may seem impossible. Some days, there are too many other threats to safety to overcome, and so we fail. If we judge ourselves harshly for this failure, then we have given ourselves one more reason why change is risky. We need to make friends with failure and have some compassion for ourselves. We need to remember that failure happens, and if we have a bad day, we can start again the next day, knowing that eventually the change will become habit or we will have learned what we needed to learn to see the benefit of the change.

GU SYNDROME

It would be short-sighted to leave a discussion of how our capacity to digest supports healthy ideation and the ability to create context for learning without touching upon the concept of Gu syndrome. The invasion of Gu or possession by Gu is a very old concept that is represented in modern times by difficult-to-treat modern disorders that disrupt digestive function such as Lyme disease and candidiasis. According to Heiner Fruehauf (Quinn and Moreland 2008), "Gu syndrome actually means that your system is hollowed out from the inside by dark *yin* forces that you cannot see." This means that part of the difficulty in the treatment of Gu is getting a diagnosis because patients with Gu often test negatively for common parasites and they have numerous symptoms that do not respond to typical Traditional Chinese Medicine treatment for digestive disorders. Patients with Gu have a combination of digestive symptoms and neurological symptoms that further reinforce the connection between the gut and the brain, and between digesting and thinking. If you are possessed by Gu, you have lost sovereignty. You are no longer in charge and therefore you are fighting for survival against an enemy you can't see and one that medical professionals can't find. Gu syndrome is usually treated with herbs, but the right acupuncture can also be helpful. Although I am not a fan of protocols, I will say that Jeffrey Yuen has given a protocol for Gu that I have found to be extremely effective. There are a number of ways to do this protocol, but I am only listing the way I typically do this. The treatment, which is called the five Gu treatment, is as follows:

Please needle in this order:

St-43/Xian Gu: Descending Valley

LI-4/He Gu: Uniting Valley

Ki-2/Ran Gu: Blazing Valley

*Sp-8/Di Ji: Earth Mechanism (not officially a Gu point)

Ki-10/Yin Gu: Yin Valley

SI-5/Yang Gu: Yang Valley

These points may be done bilaterally, but in my effort to reduce input, I usually do them unilaterally/contralaterally. With three needles on each side of the body, six needles in total:

Right St-43, left LI-4, left Ki-2, right Sp-8, left Ki-10, right SI-5

The first three points govern the transformation of food into Gu qi (St-43, LI-4 and Ki-2).

*Sp-8 wakes the Spleen up. It supports transformation and transportation (T&T) and it can be useful in restoring the ascending and descending of qi out of the middle. You can use Sp-7/Luo Gu: Leaking Valley instead if a patient has symptoms of leaky gut.

The last two points transport the Gu qi to yin and yang (Ki-10 and SI-5).

I have seen this treatment clear a greasy coat and make it normal after one application. Even though you may need more treatment to support digestion, patients are almost always thinking much more clearly after this treatment. This is essential because removing Gu makes it easier to rebuild the middle jiao and restore digestive function and increases the ability to raise clear yang to the head for cognition.

KEYS TO SELF-HELP FOR YING QI AND THE PRIMARY CHANNELS

Aside from the recommendations given earlier in this chapter, I have two things to add.

Diet, diet, diet

Change your relationship to food. Many of us are emotional eaters or over-eaters. To change our relationship to food, we may need to use some of the self-help tools recommended in the Luo-collateral section of Chapter 6. Breathe, feel your feeling and increase your circulation. Begin now to slowly do whatever you can to support healthy digestion. Small changes can have a big impact. There are many "diets" out there that claim to be the way to good health, but any one diet will not fit all. It is important that you build your own relationship with food. Pay attention to how food affects you. Pay attention to the state of your being when you decide what to eat. Are you hungry for food or hungry for comfort? Are you fueling yourself or numbing out? Put your attention on your relationship to food and nourishment and remember to have compassion for the challenges inherent in changing the habituated habits you have developed over a lifetime. The diet is important but not as important as consciously choosing what you take in.

Five spirits and symbols

The five zang organs of the Primary channel system provide residence for the five spirits, and these spirits or mental faculties support consciousness. Symbols and rituals are one of the ways we can reach those spirits and create a dialog that increases awareness. We might use the I Ching or other forms of divination such as Tarot or Mayan Oracle, not necessarily as a form of fortune-telling but as a way of allowing the unconscious mind to come forth with a subject or topic or idea that we might need to explore consciously. You could also use the Bible or the Bhagavad Gita in this fashion. You could basically use any book that inspires you, even a book of poetry. Ask for wisdom by randomly opening to a page and then try to learn something from that page. As an example of this, I did three things: I opened a random page of the I Ching, I pulled a Mayan Oracle card and I pulled a Tarot card. Here is what I received:

I Ching: Hexagram 40—Release

"The west and the south are favorable. Those with nothing to gain from going forward will win good fortune by turning back, those who have much to gain from going forward must be sure of doing well." The commentary states: "This hexagram implies activity in the face of danger, for it is activity by which danger is averted that brings release." Change is hard and scary, but embracing change and the fear associated with it is essential if we want more.

Mayan Oracle: Card 13—Universal Movement

"Thirteen touches you with the hand of unforeseen forces and radical change. It will catalyze into movement whatever resists change or is unexamined or stationary." "Drawing this number indicates that something unexpected is coming, something that may dramatically change the course of your life. You are being touched by fate, moved through identifications of self into open consciousness." I swear to you I pulled these randomly.

Tarot: 6 of Wands

"You are going to succeed; keep trying. Relationships will get better; possible journey as a leader or representative." "Efforts directed toward the arts or sciences will prove successful."

The goal is not to take these offerings as a portent of what is to come but rather to use them to begin a dialog. What becomes stirred by this communication and how do I feel about it? This is a way of giving the unconscious choices a way to surface so that the Spleen/Yi can put its attention on them and intend to bring them more fully into consciousness.

Looks as if I will be having an internal dialog about change and movement and perhaps what it might mean to let go and move on. I am sure that this communication comes about because of my intent to focus on self-preservation as a way of avoiding or resisting change.

Try this. You have nothing to lose and you may open a dialog between the conscious mind and the habituated patterns that are keeping you from being fully who you are.

A GU SYNDROME CASE STUDY

The patient was female, in her 40s, and her chief complaint was twofold: fibromyalgia and PTSD. This patient was very familiar with Chinese Medicine and had received a lot of acupuncture treatments. She came in aware of suppressed emotions and constriction in her Dai mai. Her fibromyalgia pain began around the waist and then spread out body-wide. Although the fibromyalgia pain emerged in the last few years, this patient had a history of trauma from childhood that involved family illness, sexual abuse and emotional abuse. There was no memory of birth trauma or trauma early in the first cycle of jing. Normally, I would look to the 8 EV for these types of issues, especially the Dai mai. But something about the way that this patient communicated made me want to withhold or delay diagnosis of an 8 EV pattern. During the first interview, the patient reported difficulty with focus and concentration. She had some brain fog and internal chatter that was not helpful. This patient was a student and, aside from her traumatic history, she had the challenges to her digestion that are consistent with Spleen qi deficiency. Students sit too long, think too much and frequently indulge in dietary improprieties, all of which further injure the Spleen.

Added to that, her tongue was purple with a thick yellow greasy coat and the tip was red. Her pulse was predominantly wiry, but at the depth you could feel a slippery quality if you stayed with it for a while.

I felt as though she had lost some of her sovereignty so I decided to do the five Gu treatment before making a specific diagnosis of 8 EV pathology. As mentioned earlier, Gu syndrome frequently obstructs proper diagnosis. Does she have Dai mai pathology or is the Gu making it look that way? My experience told me that I would get a clearer picture of the impact of the trauma on the 8 EV if the Gu were expelled or diminished. This protocol is a primary channel treatment that engages Ying qi to restore function.

The points were as suggested earlier in the chapter: St-43, LI-4, Ki-2, Sp-8, Ki-10 and SI-5.

I used six needles and the points were done contralaterally, as I recommended.

I saw the patient two weeks later and she reported feeling more integrated after the treatment. She had "less voices" in her head and less brain fog. What was even more important to me was her tongue went from purple to dusky (light purple, sometimes called lavender) and the greasy coat was significantly less and almost white. With one treatment, we were able to reduce the visible signs of Gu enough to see the emerging 8 EV patterns. Once we proceeded with the 8 EV treatments, the change in the fibromyalgia was pretty quick. After her first 8 EV treatment, she reported her pain was down to a "2" and she was able to work out.

During the time between the first treatment (five Gu) and the second (8 EV), she did struggle a bit with what she perceived as a flu-like condition for three weeks, but it was right before her second 8 EV treatment that she reported the tremendous relief in her fibromyalgia pain. Within a month and only two treatments (a Gu treatment and a Yang Wei treatment), she went from significant pain to almost pain-free but she had to fight for it by being sick for three of those four weeks. I believe that the battle was needed to restore her sovereignty and digestive function, and that the process was initiated by the Gu treatment. It is a little like cleaning house and saying, "Get the hell out, I am in charge of my own life." Would the Yang Wei treatment have accomplished this without the Gu treatment? I guess we will never know, but dampness, phlegm and possession are all impediments to growth. Is it not worth the time and effort to remove those impediments before attempting to restore someone's curriculum?

WHY CHOOSE A PRIMARY CHANNEL TREATMENT?

This is what you were trained to do. Typically, it is going to be your first choice. It might be easier in some ways to give you recommendations of when the Primary channels are *not* your best choice. Oh, wait, I am already doing that.

The Primary channels have no direct way to create latency. They rely on the other systems to do that for them. They rely on the Luos to either vent the pathogen to the surface or create latency in the blood far away from the organs. If the Luos fail, they rely on the Divergents to shunt the pathogen into the joints. If we experience the unbearable, then the Primary channels push the pathogen down into the Dai mai.

We choose the Primary channels not because they create latency but because they generate the post-natal resources and Ying qi circulation that is necessary to maintain that organ function. When it comes to acts of self-preservation, you may consider the Primary channels to be prudent when your patient has any of the following patterns:

- difficulty digesting (food or life or both)

- disharmony in the five Spirits (Five Element treatments can be very useful here)

- difficulty making healthy lifestyle choices (good habits are hard to build)

- poor memory that leads to learning challenges (students can benefit greatly from Primary channel treatments)

- difficulty creating context for experiences in order to learn

- possession by Gu.

Remember that we are not ruling out the fact that practitioners have been using the Primary channels plus the Du and the Ren to successfully treat all sorts of diseases for thousands of years. This is especially true if their treatments are supported with herbal prescriptions. Most everything can be treated from this level because it is in the middle and so it mediates the relationship between Wei qi and Yuan qi. However, it is important to note that treating the middle is not always the most direct or effective solution. If what you are doing is not having the desired effect, then maybe it is time to look at some of these other systems. If your resources are dwindling and you have already made the changes to your lifestyle and diet to support those resources, then maybe it is time to look elsewhere for the impediment to healing.

CHAPTER 8

THE DIVERGENT CHANNELS

C hapter 11 of the Ling Shu notes, "A beginner in acupuncture therapy should study the twelve master meridians first, and a good physician should master them in the end" (translation by Lu 2004, p.438).

It goes on to say, "Only an unskillful physician will make the mistake of thinking that the twelve master meridians are fairly easy to learn. A good physician will fully appreciate the difficulty of mastering them" (translation by Lu 2004, p.438). I have been studying and using this system for many years now and I can attest to its complexities. This system negotiates the relationship between Wei qi and Yuan qi, between inside and outside, between Self and Other. Using this system means we recognize the inherent challenges in creating a balance between how we respond externally to the world around us and who we know ourselves to be. This is no simple task because, as we have discussed in earlier chapters, human beings survive by engaging in predictable, repetitive and habituated behavior. It requires a level of unconsciousness to maintain this rote existence.

Most of us develop a reflexive coping mechanism and character style which is pre-thought or driven by the unconscious mind, and often when we engage our conscious mind, we wonder why we did what we did. The disparate needs between Wei qi (protection of the body) and Yuan qi (fulfilling our curriculum) are evidenced in this system in profound ways. It is not inaccurate to say that sometimes staying alive is at odds with who we know we are and the attempt or desire to be true to our Self. Just think of what firefighters must overcome, in terms of self-protection, to run into a burning building when all others are running away. What price do first responders pay for overriding that survival function repeatedly, and is that price worth it for the sense of satisfaction that comes from being who you really are and doing something that you are called by your spirit to do? The repeated trauma that first responders experience while doing their jobs can easily lead to Divergent pathology. This pathology can occur in any of us when we choose survival over being true to ourselves, remembering that we seldom make that choice consciously.

THE NATURE OF WEI QI AND YUAN QI

To fully appreciate the function of the Divergent system, we must understand the nature of Wei qi and Yuan qi.

Wei qi (defensive qi) circulates on the exterior of the body and protects the body from external pathogenic factors. Through its circulatory function, it warms the superficial tissues and supplies the Sinew channels, supporting locomotion. Through the sinews, it is associated with posture. The Lungs disperse Wei qi to the surface of the body and they also house the Po (Corporeal Soul). The link between these two (Wei qi and Po) manifests as physical sensation and body memory, and emotionally as mood.

As mentioned in Chapter 5, Wei qi acts as a filter for external stimulus. It is how we initially react to our external environment. The Wei qi determines if an external stimulus indicates a threat. This helps us to determine which input is going to be useful and which is not. The usefulness is usually predicated on the need for survival. This determination is not a conscious one. It is reflexive or instinctual in nature. It is pre-thought and one could say that it is pre-programmed by previous threats. We learn over time not only to recognize threat but also to anticipate it. There is a sort of learning that occurs here that comes from repeated exposure to external stimulus. Eventually, the Wei qi can learn what stimulus to ignore and it can also create a buffer that muffles the input. The Tai Yang nature of Wei qi can use fluids to dampen down the exchange between input and expression. Think of how chronic sinus congestion can make it harder to take in not only sound but also most other input.

Wei qi impacts how we take in information and experience through the senses. The level of defensiveness we have depends on how much input there is and how habituated we have become to that input. For example, if you purchase a home that is in the flight path of an airport, when you first move in, you will likely hear every plane that takes off and lands over your home. In time, Wei qi recognizes that there is no threat in the typical noise made by take-off and landing, so you stop hearing it. You stop paying attention to it, so the sound doesn't register anymore. However, if you were to hear a plane in trouble, which makes a different noise, your Wei qi would respond to that. The need for safety and survivability can set a threshold of response which determines how much input you will recognize.

At night, your Wei qi internalizes. It leaves the exterior (sinews) to receive the nourishment supplied by Ying qi in the interior. That is assuming, of course, that your Wei qi does not perceive any threat that might keep it vigilant and on the surface. What if you are homeless and sleeping in your car? Will your Wei qi feel safe enough to internalize? If it does not internalize because the threat is real, then it will be deprived of nourishment and therefore unable to do its job as well. Sleep in these circumstances is at the very least restless and frequent waking occurs. If the sense of threat is strong, sleep is impossible, and enough nights like that and you are walking around like a zombie, unable to respond effectively to any threat.

Good sleep hygiene is a way of coaxing the Wei qi inward by creating a routine and environment that projects a sense of safety.

Yuan qi is derived from jing and is closely related to the function of the Kidneys and San Jiao. It is our inherited qi and the basis of our constitution. It provides motive force for life and is the basis of organ function. As the Wei qi is linked to survival through its ability to perceive threat from the outside, the Yuan qi is linked to survival through the maintenance of organ function and survival of the species through the governance of reproduction, growth and development. Yuan qi is responsible for sustaining the functional link between the Heart and Kidney. It therefore supports the communication between body and mind through the connection between the Shen and Zhi (Spirit and Will). This means it is linked to curriculum and authenticity. It is the impetus for transformation. The motive force for change, growth and evolution is provided by Yuan qi. What if you were to be diagnosed with a condition that means you will have to change how you think about yourself? Let's say, for instance, you are told you have multiple sclerosis. Can you conceive of yourself as being the same person before the diagnosis as after? Are your beliefs about yourself the same before and after diagnosis? What if you had a near-death experience or a life-threatening injury? How might your survival and recovery affect your sense of self? What if you survived and others didn't? On a subtler level, what if in childhood you repeatedly heard phrases like "You're just too sensitive," "You'll never amount to anything," "You are an abomination," "It would have been better if you were never born"? What if you heard these things repeatedly? At what point do you change your beliefs about who you are? How long do you have to hear vitriol like this before your relationship to Self is devastatingly altered? These questions may be investigated when the Yuan qi is challenged. We like to think we know what we would do in those circumstances, but until we are faced with those choices, we can never really know.

Good health requires strong organ function. That function

is dependent on Yuan qi, and Yuan qi gives us our sense of Self. The more consciousness we have about who we are and why we are here, the more deeply we are aligned with Yuan qi. Yuan qi is the qi we use to pursue meaning and purpose in life. That does not mean to say that we cannot pursue our Destiny if we are unhealthy or if we do not have optimal function. It is about optimizing the journey by being aligned with who we are at the core and not who we become to survive. Perfection of form is not a prerequisite for consciousness, but being conscious and aligned with Self is essential if we choose to pursue meaning and purpose. We can be dying of metastatic cancer and still pursue our Destiny, but that is an almost impossible task if we are being controlled by the fear of dying. We can also respect that fear and do everything we can to beat the cancer and still accept that dying is inevitable. It becomes about how best we can use our resources to be as present as possible in the moment. The more aligned with Yuan qi we are, the more choice we have about how we will use our resources. We are capable of the fullest expression of our humanity when we are aligned with our Yuan qi and Yuan Shen.

The harmony between Wei qi and Yuan qi is a day-by-day, moment-by-moment negotiation between the need to survive and the desire to thrive. When we can strike a dynamic balance between the two, then what we take in and what we express outwardly into the world will be more genuine and reflect more authentically who we are.

MOOD VS TEMPERAMENT

Another expression of the relationship between Wei qi and Yuan qi is the level at which emotion is experienced. When emotion is experienced at the level of Ying qi, it is interactive in nature. Not only are patients often aware of what they are feeling, but they can usually tell you quite specifically what triggered their emotional response. I have already mentioned that commuting on the

405 Freeway triggers anger in me. Dealing with drivers who clearly never went to kindergarten frustrates me no end. For those of you who do not know what kindergarten is, here in the United States it is our introduction to the school system. Here we learn to share, take turns, be kind and clean up after ourselves. I have had numerous discussions with myself where I am convinced that there are many drivers on the 405 Freeway who never went to kindergarten. I know the anger is futile and I am consciously aware of what is driving it. This is anger at the Ying qi level.

If I were to awaken in the morning feeling angry or cranky for no good reason, then that would be a Wei qi type of anger. At the level of Wei qi, the anger is more like a mood. Moods tend to be less intractable, more ephemeral, and we can usually find ways to distract ourselves out of the mood. A good cup of coffee will do it for me. The ritual of brewing and then sipping the cup is a sensory delight that distracts me from any mood and lets me face the rest of the day without the weight or tension of that mood.

At the level of Yuan qi, the emotion is associated with temperament. This would be a person who has embraced anger as self. They have embodied the anger and they identify with that anger so much that they have developed deep-seated beliefs around the anger. They don't feel angry; they *are* anger. This level of anger is much more challenging to treat. It is deeply entrenched and often the person is unaware of how angry they are. Separating oneself from this kind of anger is almost like volunteering to lose a limb. It is like giving up part of yourself.

Mood, related to Wei qi, maintains our alertness. It is the aspect of our essential nature that makes us aware of the world around us. When you walk into a social setting and you feel uncomfortable, but you don't know why, that is mood. This emotional response is not directed by arousal or other triggers nor is it targeted at any one person or thing. Mood, like Wei qi, is unconscious and ephemeral. It comes and goes and is not easily explained or justified.

Temperament, on the other hand, is related to Yuan qi and is the basis of our personality or emotional tendencies. This emotional expression is influenced by aspects of nature and nurture. There is a theme to temperament that can be seen throughout our lives. We can be by nature suspicious or trusting, easy-going or defensive. We are born with a predisposition or temperament that is the basis of who we are and the framework for who we are meant to be. We may also be trained or nurtured into a different expression of temperament in childhood. This altered temperament is not who we are by nature. It is who we have become in order to survive. We may come into the world a "zen baby" with an easy-going temperament and, through neglect, abuse or a high-stress environment, we may turn into a "fussy" or "sensitive" baby that has difficulty self-soothing. If we are trained into it, we may want to release that training or trauma and return to our original Self. Our original temperament is the basis for our transcendence. It is strongly linked to our curriculum and the Self that strives for enlightenment. When we align ourselves with our temperament, the self-acceptance that occurs allows us to engage evolutionary growth in a deeper and more effective manner.

There is a directionality to these types of qi that impact how the emotion is expressed. Wei qi has an upward and outward expression. Feelings that manifest at the level of Wei qi are often short-lived or easily resolved. Yuan qi has an inward and downward inclination. Emotional states here tend to last longer. If they are not conscious or if they are habituated and accepted as Self, eventually they will result in repression, denial, numbness, fixed attitudes and diminished sensory acuity or loss of perspective. This is the place where we separate from who we are or how we feel, so that we can survive. Alignment between Wei qi and Yuan qi increases the ability to express ourselves in the most authentic manner possible in any given moment. We find the balance between survival and thriving. When the threat is serious, then survival takes precedence because if we survive, there will be time later to work towards thriving. This is the work of the Divergent system.

Also called the Jing Bie, "Distinct" or "Separate" channels, the Divergent meridians are seen as extensions of the Primary meridians and, in the context of this book, have the essential function of preserving life (Yuan qi) by creating latency. When the organs are threatened by pathogenic influence, the Divergent channels shunt the pathogen into the joints, which is the deepest aspect of the superficial areas of the body. This is where the sinews (Wei qi) and the bones (Yuan qi) meet. The pathogenic influence is held there until there are sufficient resources to either release the latency or insufficient resources to maintain the latency. This is all done to preserve life (organ function).

The Divergent system is responding to a crisis, in the form of trauma or acute and serious disease, by creating a less serious, more chronic and more slowly progressing condition. It is as if they are buying the patient time. Time to gather resources, time to gain awareness. Time to shift deeply held beliefs that may be holding them back from becoming the most authentic version of themselves. This is also time that can be used effectively to alter lifestyle and diet to support good health.

These vessels are active in the presence of a serious threat and there is clear evidence that vital substances (resources) are being used to maintain latency. Because they negotiate the relationship between Wei qi and Yuan qi, there is often a loss of sense of Self in Divergent pathology or a confusion about what is Self and what is Other.

Challenges to the Divergent system can come from the six exogenous pathogen factors (wind, cold, heat, dryness, dampness and summer-heat) or from anything that is outside, harmful to life and in the process of invading the system. Some additional disease factors may include:

- dietary improprieties or sensitivities (e.g. gluten intolerance)

- epidemic toxins (e.g. Lyme disease, Covid-19)

- environmental toxins (e.g. mold, heavy metals, pesticides).

In addition to the assault from exogenous pathogens, patients can also have this process of latency initiated by external experiences that evoke internal emotional responses (endogenous pathogenic factors) which affect a sense of Self:

- trauma, abuse, neglect

- conflict or judgment in relationships

- near-death experiences

- being diagnosed with a life-threatening or life-altering disease.

Typically, these experiences involve an interaction between Wei qi and Ying qi. As the pathogenic influences work their way past the Wei qi, Ying qi is engaged to support the Wei qi in the removal of the pathogenic factor. But if the Ying qi fails to resolve the pathogenic experience or if there is insufficient yin (blood) to hold the latency in the Luo-collaterals, Yuan qi is affected and the Divergent channels are engaged. If the patient has insufficient yin or blood prior to the invasion or trauma, Ying qi and the Luo-collaterals may be bypassed and the Divergents will be directly affected. If the pathogenic process begins in the interior (emotions) and the Primary channels or Luo-collateral system fail to expel the pathogen, then the Divergents are engaged and latency is created. This is done for the purpose of survival. Protecting the organs by sending the pathogen into the joints means increasing the chances of staying alive for longer.

For instance, if the Urinary Bladder Primary channel (Foot Tai Yang) fails to produce enough sweat or urination to dispel an exterior pathogen, the Luo system is engaged (UB-58). If the Luo system cannot successfully meet the challenge, then the pathogen moves inward, along the channel flow, towards the organs. The He-sea point (UB-40), which is also the lower meeting point of the Urinary Bladder Divergent, meets the pathogen first, trapping it in the knee joint. This isolates the pathogen safely away from the Urinary Bladder, Kidneys and Heart. In some ways, you could say that divergent pathology exists when the Luo-collateral system fails.

Because this system relies on the communication between Wei qi and Yuan qi, once the body creates the latency, it must support it by using jing. As the jing becomes overly taxed, the body will draw on other vital substances to maintain the latency. It does this in a specific order: jing first, then blood, jin (thin fluids), ye (thick fluids), qi and finally yang. An essential part of the diagnostic process is determining the state of vital substances. Which substances are in a state of repletion and which are in a state of depletion or stagnation? Treatment goals should include building resources so that the pathogen may be released or the latency can be maintained to give the patient more time.

When patients have Divergent pathology, we can see certain characteristics. The first is *chronicity*. Divergent pathology is designed to slow down the progression of disease, which means that symptoms will linger. This is not about acute joint pain from injury. It is about degeneration in the joints with chronic inflammation. Even though chronic joint pain can be devastating in terms of its impact on daily living, patients do not typically die from joint pain.

The Divergent system regulates the polarity of yin and yang, and so we usually see joint pain that is *unilateral*. In fact, it is common to see many symptoms, not just joint pain, showing up on one side. Years ago, I had an elderly patient with chronic migraines who had been treated in a school clinic with very limited success using a Zang fu diagnosis of Liver and Kidney yin deficiency with yang rising. Much of his treatment involved nourishing Liver blood and yin, anchoring yang and removing obstruction in the Gall Bladder channel. In addition to these daily migraines, he also had a benign tumor on his forehead removed. It was situated on the left Urinary Bladder channel, in the region of UB-3 and UB-4. Earlier in his life, his left kidney was removed. Although at the time I saw him his headaches were bilateral, when they began, they were typically on the left side. When latency is created, it is usually created on one side. When the vital substances that maintain the latency are depleted over time, the pain often migrates to the other side. Therefore, we see unilateral pain or *migrating pain*. These left-sided symptoms made him a very good candidate for a first confluence (Urinary Bladder/Kidney Divergent) treatment, which proved to be much more effective in treating his migraines than the typical Liver and Gall Bladder regulation. Imbalances in polarity are usually observed from left side to right side or right side to left, but they also may present as imbalances above and below, interior and exterior, or medial and lateral.

Divergent symptoms are often *intermittent*, meaning the joint pain varies in intensity and frequency. Patients with Divergent pathology often seek treatment during "flare-ups" of their chronic pain. This is typically related to the availability of resources to maintain latency. Divergent pathology will present with *consumption of resources*. The body uses vital substances to maintain latency. The longer the latency is maintained, the more the resources are depleted.

You might also see deep-seated beliefs that create specific *emotional signatures*. For instance, it is common when there is pathology in the Urinary Bladder or Kidney Divergent channels to see fear at the level of Yuan qi causing paranoia or dread of the unknown. Each Divergent confluence reflects different beliefs or responds with a different emotional expression.

We can begin to see the complexity. In order to determine which Divergent is involved in the process, we need to ascertain all of the following and more:

- How is polarity of yin and yang affected?

- Which channels are involved?

- Which organs are affected?

- What vital substances are involved in the pathology?

- What joints are involved in the latency?

- What types of movement affect the joints?

- Which cutaneous zones are congested or restricted?

- Is there a constitutional predisposition or weakness that is making the patient vulnerable?

- Are there pathological beliefs or signature emotional patterns involved in the pathology?

UPPER AND LOWER MEETING POINTS

Each Divergent channel begins in the place where it "diverges" from its associated Primary channel. This diverging process moves from Ying qi into the deeper nature of Yuan qi. This typically occurs at the major joints (hips, knees, shoulders and elbows). The lower meeting points signify where the channel "diverges." It is common for the lower meeting points to be located near the He-sea points, which may be used as substitutes for the lower meeting points. The pathways then move towards the associated paired organs, affecting the Yuan qi of those organs. They then move into the chest, affecting the Heart. This allows the system to bring a level of consciousness to the disease process, which allows for greater awareness and therefore increased choice. From the chest, the pathway rises to the upper meeting point, which is typically located in the region of the neck and face. Here the qi "emerges" to connect the Yuan qi to Wei qi. This is also the region where the Window of the Sky points are found. The Window of the Sky points may be used as substitutes for the upper meeting points. At this point, the yin Divergent channels connect to their yang paired Divergent channel and rise to Du-20/Bai Hui.

An example of this is as follows. The Urinary Bladder and Kidney Divergents separate from their Primary channels in the popliteal fossa at UB-40 and they diverge deeply into the Yuan qi level connecting with the Urinary Bladder and Kidneys. From there they rise to the Heart and then begin their journey to the surface and Wei qi to emerge at UB-10. From here, the Kidney channel joins with the Urinary Bladder channel which rises to Du-20.

Divergent pathology may exist in any chronic degenerative condition, any condition related to Wei qi deficiency or jing deficiency, structural or postural imbalances, auto-immune conditions, chronic bi syndrome. Here is a list of common conditions/diagnoses that may present as Divergent pathology:

- arthritis: chronic, degenerative, often unilateral or moving

- migraines

- chronic cystitis, especially interstitial cystitis

- visual disturbances

- hiatal hernia and reflux

- cardiovascular diseases

- diabetes and other endocrine disorders

- fibromyalgia

- endometriosis and other gynecological conditions

- osteoporosis, scoliosis, joint or muscle pain associated with posture

- chronic whiplash, body armoring, chronic muscle spasms

- respiratory problems associated with posture

- sexual dysfunction, infertility, impotence, decreased libido

- problems with teeth and/or bones

- low back pain and weakness in the knees

- premature graying of hair

- dark circles under eyes (or bags)

- persistent allergies

- environmental sensitivities

- asthma

- hypervigilance

- and many more...

This process of negotiating the relationship between Wei qi and Yuan qi can be seen in auto-immune conditions. Most auto-immune disorders are slowly progressing conditions that often are first identified by Sinew channel pathology such as joint pain, skin conditions or difficulty with locomotion. These conditions profoundly affect quality of life, but take many years to affect organ function to the point of organ failure. This means a patient might have years of ill-health that impact daily living, but they will usually be able to survive in this state for many years before the organs are damaged to the point of organ failure and death. Many auto-immune disorders are dramatically improved by lifestyle changes and by managing stress and diet. These changes support the resources that can maintain the latency or release it more effectively. What begins as a challenge to the body's defensive system (Wei qi) becomes a compensatory process where the body tries to limit the damage and slow the process of disease. The body doesn't recognize Self and an overactive immune system attacks Self. This idea of the Wei qi attacking Yuan qi because it doesn't recognize Self is commonly accepted in auto-immune conditions, but what if we can appreciate the fact that the Divergent system is working very aggressively to sustain life by maintaining latency in the joints or on the surface of the body? With this understanding, we can focus less on the eradication of symptoms and more on balancing the relationship between where the latency is trapped and the underlying resources that are essential for maintaining or releasing that latency.

ZONAL THEORY

In addition to the vital substances, diagnosis depends on the location of the disease as it relates to the Six Confluences. Basically, it is important to note which joints are affected and what type of movement or function causes or exacerbates the pain. Therefore, it is essential when using the Divergent channels to do a thorough assessment of the Sinew channels and the Cutaneous zones. The relationship between the Wei qi and Yuan qi is expressed in these six Cutaneous zones. We can see that in the way a person "holds" themselves. Their posture will indicate how their Wei qi is responding to the world outside, how it is expressing the truth of who they are (Yuan qi) or what they believe about what they are experiencing. This is a recognition of "body language." As we meet patients for the first time, it is a perfect opportunity to assess a person's posture and demeanor when they are experiencing something new. Whether conscious or not, new circumstances, experiences or situations are perceived by the Wei qi and the reptile brain as somewhat threatening because they are at the very least unpredictable. This gives us an excellent window into how the Wei qi and sinews respond to that perceived or expected threat.

Each Cutaneous zone has a certain archetypal or constitutional way that it responds to that relationship between Wei qi and Yuan qi. This can be seen in the posture, but it can also be seen in action. How a patient moves reflects their perception of the world around them and it is also an expression of what they think about themselves.

Tai Yang: Urinary Bladder and Small Intestine Divergent channels

The expression of Tai Yang is opening, upright and forward moving. The nature of Tai Yang is very directed towards moving forward in life and tackling things head-on. One could say that Tai Yang is "out there," visible and forthright. This is also true when it comes to emotional expression. Someone with a Tai Yang constitution may be very direct in expressing their emotions. There is an outward venting. A Tai Yang constitution is not holding anything in, especially if it will keep a person from moving forward. As stress, tension or stagnation increases in Tai Yang, we might see the patient develop some rigidity in the spine and in their demeanor. This might make them hold back their expression or it could make the outward expression critical and adversarial. Pathology in Tai Yang may also affect vision and perception. Patients who might benefit from looking forward become single-sighted. They may lose the ability to see their options because they develop tunnel vision, which is a narrow and overly focused state of vision. Tai Yang energy can also be seen in the arms as the Small Intestine channel allows the arms to reach out or extend into the world.

Pathology in Tai Yang often leads to back or neck pain, rigidity in the spine or repeated exterior attacks. It is common to see people who have issues with Tai Yang resemble Type A personalities. They are what I lovingly call "human doings." They are driven to keep moving, never getting to where they are headed, or if they do arrive, they quickly find a new destination. Arriving means stopping, and stopping means death. Pain associated with Tai Yang will be noticeable while walking or driving. Moving forward causes pain.

Shao Yang: Gall Bladder and San Jiao Divergent channels

The nature of Shao Yang is rotating and pivoting. This ability to move with rotation allows for flexibility and adaptability in the face of change. Rotation of the head and neck allows the Shao Yang constitution to have an expanded perspective. Peripheral vision and the ability to turn the head lets the person see their options. All of which sounds like a good thing until you get stuck in it. Stagnation in Shao Yang can often lead to frustration, depression, indecision, a wishy-washy emotional response or passive-aggressive behavior. When there is stagnation in Shao Yang, people have difficulty managing the alternating aspects of life. They have difficulty knowing when to move forward and when to stand still, or when to speak up and when to stay quiet. These patients may have conditions that reflect the inability to rotate or maintain flexibility both physically and emotionally. They often suffer from conditions such as sciatica. Shao Yang diseases also reflect the inability to maintain a balance between exterior and interior. They may have balance problems that are worse with rotating and pivoting, and their pain will be worse when twisting, turning or tilting the head. The pain is made worse in an attempt to adapt to changing environments.

Yang Ming: Stomach and Large Intestine Divergent channels

The nature of Yang Ming is closing, sitting, slowing and braking. It is about moving into yin. Yang Ming allows us to recognize when to slow down and rest. It allows us to internalize, to bring things in. This can be seen in the energy in the arms. The Hand Yang Ming channel (Large Intestine) allows us to close the hands, grasping and holding. This is not about being still. It is the active (yang) pursuit of rest. It is about engaging yang in a way that puts the brakes on. Yang Ming supports us in knowing when to sit down. Pathology is usually expressed by an increase of yang in the head, producing headaches, sinus congestion, jaw pain or other signs of heat in the head and face. You might also see pathology associated with yang deficiency. This is a result of ignoring the need for rest until the body forces the patient into stopping. These patients will report pain that is worse when standing still, bearing weight or bending forward at the hips. If the arm is involved, the patient will have difficulty gripping and holding with a straight arm. The pain is worse when we try to stop.

The yang Cutaneous zones are much larger than the yin zones, so they are easier to see and assess. The yin zones cover less surface area and are also on the medial surfaces of the body, so they are less visible. As we will see, they tend to present with less obvious changes in movement and instead present with changes in emotional expression or demeanor.

Tai Yin: Lung and Spleen Divergent channels

The nature of Tai Yin gives us the capacity to internalize and contain. When Tai Yin is overwhelmed, we begin to feel uncomfortable and a bit restless. Stillness becomes difficult. We are challenged to hold on to the experience and attempt to process it. If we cannot accomplish this, then we want to get away from the discomfort. This is the beginning of suppression. Pain here will be worse with retraction. These patients will have difficulty bringing the hands and feet towards the trunk or the knees towards the chest. Like the retraction that is caused by abdominal crunches, pain is increased by pulling inward.

Shao Yin: Heart and Kidney Divergent channels

The nature of Shao Yin maintains the connection between the Heart and Kidney and their spirits (Shen and Zhi). This relation-ship supports awareness and consciousness. When Shao Yin is challenged, we want to become unaware. The experience is painful enough that we want it to stop. Patients experience numbness, denial and repression in order to survive the challenge. Pathology here causes difficulty rotating with a bent limb. Patients will have difficulty pouring things like water from a jug; with the legs, there will be difficulty placing the ankle on the opposite thigh (rotation of the hip with a bent knee).

Jue Yin: Liver and Pericardium Divergent channels

The nature of Jue Yin (Terminal Yin or Absolute Yin) is about the ability to protect the interior. It is about the deep need for self-preservation. When Jue Yin is challenged, the need to protect the Heart (through the Pericardium) is a survival priority. This may lead to "checking out" or a state of introversion or withdrawal so complete that it leads to paralysis or total repression. This can also come as an "aha" moment or spiritual awakening in which the challenge leads to total awareness of the truth. Sometimes things become so painful that we finally get it. Immobility with constant pain is the characteristic of this pattern.

Constitutional rights

Each zone also has a "constitutional right" that is part of the make-up of our character. In the predominant elemental of a patient's constitution, this constitutional right may be viewed as a strength. The goal in the movement towards thriving is to be in alignment with that constitution as much as possible. Where the constitution is weaker, the right may seem more like vulnerability or even compensation for that weakness. Sometimes when we are stronger constitutionally in one or two zones, we manage these rights effectively. When we are weak constitutionally, embracing the right of that zone becomes part of our curriculum. The rights are as follows:

> **Tai Yang:** The right to *act*. This is the right to initiate movement. The right to move towards something. Tai Yang allows us to put one foot in front of the other and act in a way that is in alignment with our destiny or curriculum. Weakness in Tai Yang may lead to ineffective movement or movement that is not well directed. We may even find it difficult to engage the drive to move at all. We embrace the right of Tai Yang every time we put our will into action. Do something.

Shao Yang: The right to *decide*. This is the right to choose. We have the right to decide for ourselves what will serve us. When there is a weakness in Shao Yang, we may become wishy-washy. We may be easily discouraged or find it difficult to make decisions. We embrace this right when we muster up the courage needed to choose. You decide.

Yang Ming: The right to *demand/need*. This is the right to ask for what we want or need without feeling guilty, weak or dependent. When there is weakness in Yang Ming, we will find it difficult to ask for help. We may feel as if asking for help is a failure, or we may be worried that if we ask, someone will say no. We embrace this right when we risk the vulnerability it takes to ask for help. Just ask.

Tai Yin: The right to *embrace/accept*. This is the right to receive without embarrassment or obligation and enjoy the gift. It is the right to embrace our worthiness, our value. When we have a weakness in this Tai Yin constitution, we may not be able to receive graciously. We may feel embarrassed by the gift or even a compliment. To support this right is an act of self-esteem. I am worthy.

Shao Yin: The right to *measure/impart value*. This the right to acknowledge what is important to us. It is the right to set priorities based on our own set of values. When there is a weakness in constitutional Shao Yin, we are unable to place value on our needs or our beliefs. This, in turn, means that we are unable to place a value on ourselves and our time. Embracing this right means setting limits and getting clear on your own standards. This is important to me.

Jue Yin: The right to *occupy*. This is the right to exist, to be, to take up space in the world without fear. It is the right to occupy your place in the world without justification. When there is a weakness in the constitution of Jue Yin, we feel as though we must earn our right to exist. We must prove to the world that it is right and good that we are here. We embrace this right when we fully understand that we do not have to earn our right to be here. We need not apologize for being here. It is enough that we exist. I am, we are.

When there is pathology affecting the Tai Yang Cutaneous zone, the patient will have difficulty expressing themselves effectively through action. When the pathology affects Shao Yang, patients will have difficulty seeing their options and making decisions. When the pathology is in Yang Ming, patients will exhaust themselves because they cannot easily ask for help. When there is Tai Yin pathology, patients tend to find it difficult to be well contained. This leakiness is accompanied by a resistance to receiving help when it is offered, even if it is just a hug. Pathology in the Shao Yin zone will make it difficult to connect with what is important to the Heart and Kidney axis, which makes it challenging to set limits and maintain sovereignty. In Jue Yin zone pathology, existence is painful, and the world is a scary and hostile place.

ELEMENTAL ARCHETYPES OF THE DIVERGENT CHANNELS

The Six Confluences also have Five Element associations and the characteristics of these constitutions can often be seen in physical gestures and also in specific dispositions or reflexive modes of response.

Water

The archetypal motto of water is "adapt or die." As a river returns to the sea, the water must find its way around obstacles that might stop its flow. If the water stops, it becomes stagnant and dies. Life will find a way.

Gestures: Facial gestures and movement of the limbs are fluid or wavy.

Urinary Bladder: The yang aspect of water has the inclination to plow through obstacles and to be in charge. It runs on the principle of lead, follow or get out of the way, but keep moving. This archetypal nature is often associated with strong feelings that may be unexpressed but can easily be felt by others, like an undertow in the ocean.

Kidney: The yin aspect of this archetype is typically associated with very sensitive people who tend to be introverted, often pursuing spiritual paths and having a strong need for an inner sanctuary. They are like the expression "still waters run deep."

Wood

The archetypal nature of wood is directed, goal-oriented and idealistic.

Gestures: The pioneering impulse of Wood can be seen in gestures as an impulse to move or express in the moment. These people are always ready to act. Like the nature of a seed sprouting, breaking through the soil and reaching up for the sunlight.

Gall Bladder: The yang aspect of wood wants to lead. It wants to be noticed for being high-achieving. It wants to stand out. This type can frequently be heard saying, "I have a plan for that."

Liver: The yin aspect of Wood supports visions of the future. It is the ability to see potential or the possibility of a future. Sometimes the vision can be unrealistic because it is based on looking backward. The yin aspect of Wood appreciates change. It is focused on growing and is willing to embrace change to evolve. Like the seasonal impact on flowers and trees, the Wood soul looks forward to the newness of spring, the abundant heat of summer, the dying and restful energy of fall and the hibernation and restoration of winter. The Wood nature of the Liver is looking forward to the cyclic change that is life. Keep growing.

Earth

The archetypal nature of Earth is focused on power. Since the Earth element governs digestion, which is the source of power in the body, we see the Earth element establishing a relationship to power. Earth constitutions tend to be strong-willed.

Gestures: Because the Earth is the central element, gestures associated with Earth come from a grounded state and are therefore slow and balanced.

Stomach: The yang aspect of Earth likes to mediate and enjoys engaging others. It can, in its enthusiasm to mediate, overpower others and dominate in relationships.

Spleen: The yin aspect of Earth is more likely to be accommodating. The yin nature of Earth seeks to comfort others, and if others are not happy, it tends to be self-critical. This often leads to an overreaction to criticism, as people with this aspect of Earth are already harder on themselves.

Fire

The archetypal nature of Fire is volatile and combustible. These people are not necessarily prone to angry outbursts like Wood imbalances, but rather they have quick and easy access to their emotions. They like the "spark" that ignites in engaging others. They tend to be very people-oriented.

Gestures: The quick and combustible nature of Fire makes gestures abrupt and jerky.

Small Intestine: The yang aspect of Imperial Fire is intellectual and thrives on challenges. This aspect of Fire loves a meeting of the minds.

Heart: The yin aspect of Imperial Fire is charismatic and hypnotic. This aspect of Fire loves the allure of relationship.

San Jiao: The yang aspect of Ministerial Fire is linked to the deep knowing of Yuan qi and is associated with intuition and creativity.

Pericardium: The yin aspect of Ministerial Fire is sentimental and holds on to the past. This constitution likely has a box of saved treasures like birthday cards from their childhood.

Metal

The Metal archetype is about the need for order in the world. These people tend to be more image-oriented because they appreciate that beauty is a representation of that order.

Gestures: The orderliness of Metal means that gestures are typically evenly paced and purposeful.

Large Intestine: The yang nature of Metal prefers to have all their ducks in a row. They tend to be level in demeanor, especially if all the baby ducks comply.

Lung: The yin aspect of Metal doesn't multitask. They prefer to focus on one thing at a time. There is a mindfulness in that focus that cannot happen when they are expected to multitask.

This elemental and archetypal nature is deeply reflected in how we hold ourselves in the moment. Someone with a Metal constitution will naturally hold themselves in a different way than someone with a Fire constitution. This, in turn, affects our ability to stay present in the moment. Appreciating your elemental nature allows you to align yourself with that nature and express yourself more authentically. If you can release the soft tissue, changing the posture, you can change the awareness of the moment. Re-posturing can change the way we think, and it can positively impact our constitution. Freeing the structure through the sinews can also support an individual's ability to embrace the weaker aspects of their constitution and evolve.

Through the Divergent channels, we are releasing the Wei qi and sinews to support the Yuan qi and constitution. Since Yuan qi is disseminated by Wei qi via the Sinew channels, we can see that trauma or abuse that reaches the level of Yuan qi can be somatized into the musculo-skeletal system by the Divergents in order to protect the Zang fu. This attack on Yuan qi engages the Divergent channels to create latency in the joints which disrupts range of motion and movement potential. Thus, the impact of trauma can often be seen in the posture or our capacity for easy movement. When we have experienced trauma that affects our sense of Self, the Wei qi and sinews learn to brace in preparation for the next assault. Here we may also see the creation of body memory. To survive the violation of trauma, we often store the pathogenic aspect of that trauma in the soft tissues as a body memory. This allows us to suppress the emotions associated with the experience of the trauma, making us less conscious of that experience so that we can try to move forward after the trauma. This is useful for survival purposes, but we must also recognize that the body never forgets. It requires a tremendous effort and abundant resources to maintain that body memory and keep it in the superficial tissues far, far away from the conscious mind. The cost of continued survival can be very steep. Movement that is braced and waiting for the next assault is never free and spontaneous. It is often rigid and usually painful. Even though it gives us the gift of time, it robs us of the ability to move in the world in a way that truly reflects who we are.

THE CONFLUENCES

I highly recommend when studying the functions of this system that you have the images of the pathways, found in many textbooks, in front of you while reading. Being able to see the pathway while learning the functions and indications helps to make the theory more sensible and concrete. Much of the function is based on where the channel goes. In this section, we will explore the key points of each confluence and the indications for its use. Each of the confluences has a yang and a yin pathway. These can be treated together or each Divergent can be treated separately. Having the images in front of you while we explore each confluence will anchor the connection between function and location. This may help you to decide whether to treat the confluence as a whole or to choose between the yang or yin Divergent.

Confluence 1: Urinary Bladder and Kidney

The first confluence includes the Urinary Bladder and Kidney Divergent channels. This confluence uses jing to maintain latency. It may seem a little counterintuitive that the substance we consider most precious would be used before all other substances to create and maintain latency. Jing is indeed precious, and because it is so valuable, we bank it. We keep a healthy reserve. We store it in the Kidneys for emergencies so that it may support growth, development and procreation. It is meant to be drawn upon for issues related to survival. For instance, when a person experiences shock, the qi and blood scatters. This disruption in the qi mechanism can lead to death, but one of the reasons why most people do not die of shock is the easy access to jing to maintain organ function. The hallmark of the Divergent system is latency created when Yuan qi is threatened; this is a survival issue and therefore jing is the appropriate mediumship for latency. Of course, the first confluence includes the Kidneys where the jing is stored, so the system doesn't have to go very far to access it.

The first confluence diverges from the Primary channels in the popliteal fossa at UB-40 and emerges in the nape of the neck in the region of UB-10. Along its pathway, it connects with and influences the anus, the Urinary Bladder, the Kidneys, the Heart and the brain. It also connects with the Dai mai through Du-4 and UB-23. In fact, the posterior aspect of the Dai mai emerges from the Kidney Divergent at the level of Du-4. The deep connection to Yuan qi strengthens the relationship between the Urinary Bladder and Kidney for chronic patterns involving either or both organs. This link with the organs of the lower burner and the connection to the anus and Dai mai means that this confluence has a very powerful impact on consolidation in the lower burner. It governs how we hold things in and how we let things go through urination, defecation and sexual function. The Urinary Bladder pathway flows through the Heart, strengthening the relationship between the Heart and Kidney, which is essential to maintain the balance between Fire and Water. Add the connection to the brain and you have a system that can be used effectively to treat neurological and psycho-emotional patterns.

The Wei qi aspect of this system homes to the chest, specifically the Pericardium loop (UB-15, GB-22, Ren-17). Patients with pathology in the first confluence frequently present with muscle pain or tension in the chest and hypochondriac region ("ring around the chest"). In the creation of latency, the Urinary Bladder draws the pathogenic factor towards the shoulder at SI-10. Because of this, there may be restricted range of motion in the shoulder. The Shao Yin (Kidney) aspect of this confluence can produce Wei qi restriction in the region of the throat (Ren-23). The pathway of this confluence supports and regulates the ascending and descending of qi in the head and along the spine. Through this function, we are able to treat many chronic musculo-skeletal problems. Indications for the use of the first confluence are:

- chronic joint pain (especially low back and knee pain)

- spinal problems: spinal tumors, scoliosis, kyphosis, vertebral stenosis

- palpitations: anxiety, cardiac rhythm problems, hypertension, hypotension

- wind: chronic allergies, environmental sensitivities, neurological disorders

- symptoms in the head: headaches (occipital, hypertensive and heat-related), chronic sinusitis, tooth pain or decay, nasal polyps

- Wei qi disorders: chronic swollen glands, nodules, sore throat, throat tumors

- Dai mai disorders: chronic cystitis, vaginal discharge and diarrhea (damp-heat), genital herpes, intercostal neuralgia

- any chronic Kidney pattern: especially those conditions related to an inability to consolidate in the lower burner or yin deficiency with yang rising.

Signature emotion: Paranoia, chronic dread of the unknown.

Confluence 2: Gall Bladder and Liver

This confluence uses blood to maintain latency. In the process of invasion from exterior to interior, Shao Yang may be considered next in line because it is half exterior and half interior. The implication is that jing has been excessively used in the first confluence and in the second confluence the next substance readily available is blood. The second confluence takes blood from the front-mu points and the Dai mai. The confluence diverges from the Primary channels in two places. The Gall Bladder diverges in the lateral thigh (GB-30) and the Liver diverges on the dorsum of the foot (St-42). This diverging point also connects the Liver

Divergent with the Chong mai (Sea of Blood). The confluence emerges in the region of the lateral canthus (GB-1). Along the pathway, it connects with the Gall Bladder, Liver, Heart and eyes. It connects with the Chong mai and the Pericardium loop. Its pathway supports the genitalia, diaphragm and the rectus abdominis, giving the practitioner a further connection to the Dai mai through the ancestral sinews. This confluence connecting the Gall Bladder to the Liver allows the Liver to influence the lateral aspects of the head and eyes. It regulates the ascending and descending of qi to and from the head. The connection between the Gall Bladder and Liver strengthens the ability to treat pathology in the genital region (especially dampness).

The Wei qi aspect of this confluence is "rooted" in the lower burner. The Wei qi zone is in the region of the Dai mai, "ring around the waist" (GB-25 to Ren-3/2). The Gall Bladder draws the pathogenic factor to the San Jiao channel in the region of the jaw. The Jue Yin (Liver) aspect may present with Wei qi congestion in the lateral aspect of the breast (Pc-1). Patients who have latency created in this confluence may have:

- osteoporosis (hip and pelvis), difficulty rotating the hips

- impotence or excessive libido

- uterine fibroids or other gynecological conditions related to blood stasis or dampness accumulating in the Dai mai

- splenomegaly/hepatomegaly (especially associated with blood stasis pain)

- flank and chest pain: intercostal neuritis, zoster/shingles, hypochondriac pain and distension due to emotional constraint, anxiety

- throat problems: plum pit, dry throat, hoarse voice, laryngitis

- one-sided headaches including migraines

- visual problems (especially spot in the visual field at GB-1)

- alternating fever and chills (Shao Yang disorders), malaria.

Signature emotion: Manic-depression. When the San Jiao and Dai mai are involved, there is a need to collect clutter.

Confluence 3: Stomach and Spleen

This confluence uses thin fluids (jin) to help maintain latency. We are moving from outside to inside, from Tai Yang to Shao Yang and then Yang Ming. Yang Ming is fully interior. The Stomach is the source of post-natal fluids and its function provides the thin fluids for latency. This confluence diverges in the region of the thigh (St-30) connecting to the Spleen, Stomach, Pericardium and Heart. It emerges in the throat and rises to the face and eye at UB-1. The yin and yang aspects of the confluence unite in the pelvic region to connect with the Chong mai. The Wei qi expresses through a zone in the region of the neck as a "ring around the collar" (St-12 to Ren-22 to Du-14). The Stomach Divergent draws the pathogenic factor towards the clavicle. Tension can be found where the muscles of the neck attach to that region. The Tai Yin (Spleen) aspect will present with tension in the neck (St-9 to LI-18). This confluence enhances the ability of the Stomach and Spleen to strengthen the legs, especially the thighs. It also has a connection to the Chong mai and the Sea of Nutrition (Ying) that makes it useful in the treatment of chronic digestive disorders. The Spleen Divergent passes through Ren-23 and therefore strengthens the Spleen's connection to the tongue. Indications for use:

- digestive disorders (especially those due to Stomach and Spleen disharmonies)

- inner thigh pain

- pelvic pain

- lower abdominal pain

- hernias (hiatal and inguinal)

- breast problems

- throat problems (esophageal constriction)

- dental pain (especially front teeth)

- nasal polyps, sinus conditions

- eye pressure and pain (including glaucoma).

Signature emotion: Lack of will to do anything for oneself but will do anything for others. It also may present emotionally as a lack of internal drive/chronic boredom.

Confluence 4: Small Intestine and Heart

This confluence uses thick fluids (ye) to support latency. These denser fluids serve to lubricate the joints and sensory orifices. They are also found in the cerebral-spinal fluids. As the thin fluids become less and less available, the Divergent system now begins to access the denser fluids that are less mobile. Endocrine fluids will be affected by this draw. This confluence diverges in the region of the Pericardium loop at GB-22/Pc-1. It passes through the axilla (Ht-1) and into the chest, affecting the Heart, where the yang and yin aspects unite at Ren-17. Descending branches pass through all three burners to Ren-4 where the confluence intersects with the Small Intestine organ and the ascending branches pass through the cheeks to affect the eyes at UB-1. Since the Small Intestine is Tai Yang, Wei qi constriction occurs in the Pericardium loop ("ring around the chest"). The Shao Yin (Heart) constriction can be found at Ren-23, producing a tightening sensation in the throat. The movement through all three burners allows this Divergent to regulate the polarity of fluid imbalances (endocrine fluids and blood). It gathers Wei qi to prevent leakage and hemorrhage. It is therefore very useful in the treatment of bleeding disorders and hormonal imbalances. It supports cardiovascular health by bringing blood to the head, connecting the Heart and brain. Increased blood flow to the head also supports sensory organ function. Indications include:

- stroke, dizziness, faintness on exertion

- poor memory, insomnia

- hormonal imbalances

- lymph and axillary swelling

- fibrocystic breasts

- fluid imbalances

- digestive dysfunction

- bleeding in the upper body.

Signature emotion: Rationalization or obsession with the rational. Rationalization is a way of justifying one's experience. If you are unable to rationalize, then you must trivialize, generalize or exaggerate the problem. Patients with pathology in this confluence may also experience serious self-loathing; they would rather be someone else. Caught in self-loathing with an inability to rationalize one's experience, one might be forced into a state of dissociation to survive. Dissociative identity disorder (DID) may present in this confluence. This is also the place where Shadow work occurs. Patients have an opportunity to get to know the dark side of Self.

Confluence 5: San Jiao (Triple Burner) and Pericardium

This confluence uses qi to maintain latency after fluids are depleted. Because the San Jiao is both the avenue of Yuan qi and the official in charge of fluid metabolism, it uses qi to mobilize dampness for maintaining latency. It is now drawing on pathological fluids (dampness) because the healthy fluids are no longer easily available. This is a much more desperate creation of latency. We are running out of time and resources. The confluence diverges in the abdomen at Ren-12 and emerges on the throat, behind the ear at SJ-16. The San Jiao Divergent begins at Du-20 and the Pericardium begins in the flank at GB-22. They unite in the chest at Ren-17 and affect all three burners, the Pericardium and the retro-auricular region of the head. The Wei qi zone affected by the Divergent is Shao Yang and congestion is found in the region of the Dai mai ("ring around the pelvis"). The San Jiao draws the pathogenic factor towards GB-12. The Jue Yin aspect of the Pericardium may create tension in the region of Pc-1. The neck and the pelvis must be freed for treatment of this Divergent to be effective. This can be done by using superficial modalities such as gua sha, cupping and tui na, or one could also use the Window of the Sky and Doorway to the Earth points in the treatment. Treating this confluence is about the ability to keep the fluids balanced in the San Jiao. Regulating exocrine and endocrine fluids maintains the dynamic balance of fluids, which then manages heat. When latency is lost in this confluence, the first four areas affected are the chest, the neck, the throat (and sensory orifices) and the bones. These are common areas where cancer originates, especially if the latent pathogen is a heat toxin. It might be helpful for this purpose to think of cancer as a perversion or mutation of Yuan qi. Indications for use:

- imbalances in fluid pairings: for example, cold-damp above with yin deficiency below

- excess phlegm, fluids, nasal discharge

- Shen disturbances associated with heat affecting yin (empty heat and blood heat)

- chest pain, palpitations, insomnia (heat and phlegm)

- wind

- organ failure

- organ inflammation

- unresponsive infections.

Signature emotion: The Pericardium is the Heart protector or the Heart constrictor. The conflict is the ability to bear the unbearable while allowing others to love us. This conflict can result in either egocentricity or lack of Self, delusions, mania, stuttering, jealousy or possessiveness.

Confluence 6: Large Intestine and Lung

This is the final confluence. It is the end stage. At this point, qi is nearly lost and the confluence uses yang to attempt to maintain latency. Patients present with jing deficiency and cold symptoms. Movement and heat are compromised, so the pulses will be slow, and the tongue may be blue or purple. The patient is running out of time and resources. The Large Intestine begins at LI-15, moves towards DU-14 (six yang meeting), then returns to the anterior chest at St-12 where it diverges. It has three branches that affect the axilla, trunk and neck, and it emerges at LI-18. The Lung Divergent descends from Lu-1 into the chest and Lungs, and ascends through the clavicle and emerges in the neck at LI-18 and rises to GB-8. This confluence unites at St-12 in the clavicular region and connects to the Large Intestine and Lungs. The Large Intestine Divergent uses yang in a last-ditch attempt to maintain latency and the yin Divergent (Lung) has little to offer, so it is advisable to do everything possible to maintain the latency to preserve life.

Efforts are also made to support the expelling of pathogenic fluids since the Lungs cannot expel, the Spleen cannot transform and the Kidney cannot dissipate due to the loss of yang. Du-14 is a pivotal point in this process. Du-14 is six yang meeting and it allows the Primary channels to access the Yang of the Du mai. The Large Intestine Divergent has a Yang Ming Wei qi zone. Tension or congestion will be found in the "ring around the collar." The Lung's Wei qi zone is Tai Yin and will be blocked between St-9 and LI-18. Indications for its use include:

- unilateral pain or swelling in the shoulder

- chronic rebellious qi of Lung or Stomach, running piglet

- glandular swelling (salivary and clavicular), goiter

- hair loss (jing cannot traverse the neck)

- serious intestinal diseases

- chronic respiratory diseases

- cardiac or respiratory failure

- seizures.

Signature emotion: "Law and order" morality. Patients have an overblown sense of justice or vindictiveness. One might see psychopathic tendencies or vigilantism, where patients take the law into their own hands and feel justified in doing so. This may look like chaos in search of order.

The goal of the Divergent channels is the healthy release of stored somatic stagnation. When using these vessels, we must pay attention to body language and postural changes. We need to be able to observe where the life force is stuck or over-expressed.

Attention to limits in movement or limits in the patient's ability to react is also important. The armoring that limits movement must be released to fully release the emotional stagnation. The Divergent channels can help us fulfill our destiny or at the very least help us to see our resistance to our destiny. In pursuit of our destiny, our expressions and actions must be aligned with the deepest truth of who we are. The Divergent meridians can help us achieve that alignment. They give us the time we need to gain awareness and perspective so that we can choose to do whatever is necessary to realign ourselves in a way that is more authentic.

TREATING THE DIVERGENT CHANNELS

When deciding to treat the Divergents, you must decide whether you want to release the latency or help the patient to maintain the latency. This is typically decided based on the patient's resources. If a patient is strong and has sufficient resources, you can release the latency. If they are weak or their resources are compromised, then it is advised to help the patient maintain the latency until they can gather the necessary internal or external resources to support the release.

When in doubt, support the latency; releasing the latency in a patient who has insufficient resources may cause a healing crisis.

The release or maintenance of the latency may be accomplished with needle technique. Releasing the latency requires a technique that is shallow-deep-shallow (S-D-S). The needle is first inserted superficially, taken deep and then brought up close to the surface and left in the superficial tissue. This directness brings the pathogen up to the surface for venting.

To maintain the latency, do the opposite: deep-shallow-deep (D-S-D). This technique holds the latency and supports the resources by telling the body it is not yet time to let go. Hold on a little longer.

THE UPPER AND LOWER MEETING
POINTS OF THE SIX CONFLUENCES

When you decide which confluence you want to treat, you will need to let the qi know where to "diverge" into Yuan qi and where to "emerge" so that Yuan qi can connect to Wei qi. The lower meeting points are located in an area where the qi can be directed more deeply, and the upper meeting points are located in an area where the qi can easily surface or emerge. You can think of them as signposts that direct the qi to rectify the relationship between Yuan and Wei qi.

Table 8.1 Upper and lower meeting points

Confluences	Upper meeting point (Wei qi)	Lower meeting point (Yuan qi)
UB/Ki	UB-10	UB-40
GB/Lv	GB-1	Ren-2
St/Sp	UB-1 (St-9)	St-30
SI/Ht	UB-1	GB-22 (Pc-1)
SJ/Pc	SJ-16	St-12 (Ren-22, GB-22)
LI/Lu	LI-18	St-12

If you decide to use a single Divergent, rather that the confluence, then you will want to add an opening point to the treatment. In some cases, these are the same as the lower meeting points. These points indicate where the individual channel "diverges." They basically instruct the body to focus on either the yin or the yang channel, not both.

Table 8.2 Opening points

Confluence	Yang	Yin
UB/Ki	UB-40	Ki-10
GB/LV	GB-30	L-5

cont.

Confluence	Yang	Yin
St/Sp	St-30	SP-12
SI/Ht	SI-10	HT-1
SJ/Pc	Du-20	GB-22
LI/Lu	LI-15	LU-1

ASSESSING THE ZONES

Each of the six confluences has an area or band where the Wei qi homes or gathers. These areas are typically palpated for tenderness or restriction. These are also areas that need to be cleared or opened prior to or during treatment. You can do this with cupping, gua sha, massage or adding needles in the area to free the qi.

Tai Yang: Palpate the ring around the chest (Pericardium loop, diaphragm).

Shao Yang: Palpate the ring around the pelvis (Dai mai).

Yang Ming: Palpate the ring around the collar (where the neck attaches to the trunk).

Tai Yin: Palpate the thyroid area (between St-9 and LI-18).

Shao Yin: Palpate the throat near the base of the tongue (Ren-23).

Jue Yin: Palpate the lateral aspect of the breast area (Pc-1). If you are uncomfortable palpating the breast tissue, check for tension in the flank, below the breast or lower ribs, in the tissue surrounding the breast. Palpate GB-22, Sp-21, St-18 or Lv-14. Tension near these points will reflect the resistance at Pc-1.

Additional points:

Jing-well points: These are added for S-D-S treatments as an exit route for the sinew involved. These are used when you are trying to release the latency.

Midline points: (Usually Du-20) encourages Wei qi to cross the midline, typically pointed towards the side that has the jing-well point. You can use any midline point and direct it slightly towards the side of pain.

Ah Shi points: Needle this point if gua sha doesn't relieve the tenderness or if you want to use needles to free the sinews in a specific area.

Yuan level points: Back-shu, front-shu, Yuan-source, He-sea, Influential points, mu points.

Xi-cleft points: Although they are not yuan level, they can be used for leakage or lost latency.

For Divergent treatments to be the most successful, you need to be sure that the Wei qi is open and circulating. Check the appropriate Wei qi zone for your treatment and:

- Needle, gua sha, cup, plum-blossom or massage the zone for musculo-skeletal release.

- Ensure the Fu organs are open for elimination, especially the bowels (St-25 is useful).

- Scars can block Wei qi; treat before or concurrently.

- You can also have the patient use castor oil packs for scarring between treatments at home.

KEYS TO SELF-HELP FOR WEI QI, YUAN QI AND THE DIVERGENT CHANNELS

Self-help for Wei qi can be found in Chapter 5. To address the Yuan qi, try the following.

Breathe

This type of breathing is deep into the belly and then we exhale until there is no breath left. We expand the belly as we breathe deeply into the lower Dan Tian to the place where we are sourced. This is the place where Yuan qi emerges from Ming Men, the Gate of Vitality. It is the place that anchors our spirit and our breath. On the exhale, we empty the breath completely, and as we do this, we empty the body of that which no longer serves our humanity. We exhale completely, emptying our cup and sharing our life force with the world around us. When we exhale fully, emptying the lungs, we open ourselves to be filled with the life force of the Universe in a way that reminds us of how connected we are. When you first start to do this, you may feel a little dizzy or light-headed after a few deep breaths. Start slowly with just a few deep breaths and build your way up. You will derive great benefit from just a few of these breaths.

Find stillness

We can do this with meditation or by practicing mindfulness, which facilitates our ability to be as fully present in the moment as possible. When we are still and fully present in the moment, we are more deeply connected to the truth of who we are. Spending time in nature can be very helpful here. For some of us, it may be as simple as stopping for a few moments each day to have a cup of lovingly prepared tea and contemplate our place in the universe. This stillness can also be found watching the waves hit the shore or the sun set beyond the horizon.

Engage the Observer

The Observer is that aspect of Self that is not injured by life's challenges. From this place, we can see our predicaments more objectively and we have more choice. This is simply about choosing to take a step back and watch ourselves, without judgment, as we try to negotiate those life challenges. When we are trying to free up an old pattern, we have to see ourselves in it. It is a little like asking an alcoholic to give up their addiction when they cannot yet see it as a problem. Engaging the Observer allows us to bring our attention to the problem and intend for it to be different. This is not about judging ourselves. This is about seeing ourselves with a sort of compassionate detachment. Once we can see the reality of what is, we can address the problem and ask for help.

A DIVERGENT CHANNEL CASE STUDY

This is the same patient I wrote about in Chapter 6. He is now in his 70s. If you live long enough and your life is challenging enough, you may eventually create latency at all levels. This patient had latency created in Wei, Ying, Yuan and jing—all necessary to survive. After being treated for some of the things we previously discussed, the patient reported one-sided pain in the left shoulder in the region of SI-10. The pain was intermittent and often radiated down into the arm from the area just medial to the joint near the scapula. In the past, he had also complained of low back pain and he had a history of kidney stones. This kidney history and his life-long fear to the point of paranoia was why I chose the first confluence rather than one of the last three confluences to treat the shoulder pain. Chiropractic treatment to release fascial adhesions provided temporary relief, but eventually the pain would return. As a reminder, this patient had a long history of addiction and abusive relationships.

The first Divergent treatment began with moxa on the left shoulder, with a focus on the area of the shoulder near SI-10. The Urinary Bladder Divergent draws Wei qi to this area. I chose moxa instead of cupping or gua sha because the area of pain was not hot or red and the patient had both Kidney yin and yang deficiency.

Because of this patient's age, thinness and yin deficiency, I chose to focus on supporting the latency rather than pushing for a release. You could do that with a D-S-D needle technique or also with needle order. I chose to minimize needle stimulation and set my intent for supporting latency by starting at the head where the Wei qi expresses and moving towards the feet, moving towards Yuan qi. The needles were inserted in the following order:

Du-20: Inserted angled towards the feet.

UB-10: Upper meeting point (Wei qi). Inserted perpendicular for safety but with the intention of moving the Wei qi towards Yuan qi.

SI-10: Bilaterally because both were tender. Angled slightly downward towards the feet.

UB-43: Back-shu of the Pericardium to address the chronicity of the condition and to free up the Wei qi tension in the Pericardium loop. Also needled slightly downward.

Du-9: To open the diaphragm and free up the Pericardium loop.

UB-23: Back-shu of Kidneys (you could choose Du-4 or even UB-52 instead). These points are all on the posterior portion of the Dai mai. Needles were angled down.

UB-40: Lower meeting point (Yuan qi) to complete the Divergent. Slight downward angle of needle.

This treatment was repeated three times with one or two small changes, every two weeks, and after the third treatment the shoulder pain was gone and the paranoia and fear were much less invasive.

I have been treating this patient, on and off for a while, and although he definitely wants to feel better, I don't think that is why he comes to see me. He is very aware of the weight of his history. I believe he is using the acupuncture treatments as a way to continue to increase insight and awareness. In his work, he is helping others to heal old wounds and I think he knows that when you are responsible for holding the space for someone's awakening, you had better be working on your own. He is a sad soul, and I mean that in the best way. His heart has been broken many times and he is not afraid to accept and feel the loss. That makes him an excellent companion as his client's journey into their dark night of the soul. The upsides of investing in loss are compassion for the suffering of others and a deep appreciation for quiet moments of contentment. As he is able to engage the Observer with compassionate detachment for himself, he is also able to hold that space for others.

WHY CHOOSE A DIVERGENT TREATMENT?

The Divergent system is about finding a way to give a patient more time to deal with life-altering events. It is about having a system that is designed to create a less devastating, more slowly progressing illness that increases the chance of survival rather than being overwhelmed by experiences we are unable to process. The key to choosing a Divergent is chronicity. We need to be able to see how an event or experience diverted the course of someone's life. We need to recognize the ill-ease caused by that diversion. The imbalance between Wei qi and Yuan qi is manifest in polarity imbalances. Symptoms will be unilateral or migrating. Because the latency depends on sufficient resources, and resources fluctuate based on stress and lifestyle choices, we also see intermittent symptoms. Patients with Divergent pathology have "flare-ups" of symptoms. Some of the acts of self-preservation that warrant the need for Divergent response are:

- shock

- near-death experiences

- devastating medical diagnosis (cancer, heart disease, stroke, dementia)

- abuse that alters our sense of Self (physical, emotional or spiritual, such as cult experiences)

- virulent pathogens (Covid-19, vector diseases that produce chronic and lingering symptoms after the infection subsides, such as Lyme disease)

- chronic life-altering digestive diseases (Crohn's, inflammatory bowel disease, digestive malignancy).

What we are looking for here is disease that appears to be more superficial (sinews)—disease that affects daily function but is not critical. This is disease that is focused on managing symptoms rather than taking heroic measures. What we will see is patients struggling to manage their lives but not necessarily beset by fears of dying. These conditions might actually make us think of the sinews but they will have a deeper and more chronic presentation. We may also be lucky enough to have patients tell us that the symptoms began shortly after some life-altering event. For instance, it is not uncommon to hear the stories of breast cancer patients including a history of great loss, 12–18 months prior to their diagnosis. We also need to be aware that Divergent pathology may occur after all of the other systems fail. In that sense, there may not be one life-altering event. What we may see instead is repeated attacks on the sense of Self that over time leads to the "straw that broke the camel's back." The precipitating event may seem rather small, but when you add that to a history of events that erode the sense of Self, the picture becomes clearer. When the patient is suffering from chronic degenerative pain in the superficial regions of the body and Primary channel treatments have failed to produce the desired results, investigate the Divergent system.

CHAPTER 9

THE EIGHT EXTRAORDINARY VESSELS

As I write this chapter on the Eight Extraordinary Vessels (8 EV) during the Covid-19 pandemic of 2020, I am reminded that some experiences in life are so big, so devastating, so life-altering that we must re-examine every part of how we are living. If ever there was a clear example of evolutionary stress, this pandemic is it. Because of the global spread of this tiny but highly contagious virus, we were asked to reconsider our lives in dramatic and tremendously uncomfortable ways.

In the USA, once the spread of the virus became devastatingly obvious, we were warned to change our way of existence. We were advised to change the way we approach hygiene. We were told that the virus was highly contagious, and the death rate appeared to be much higher than is typical for seasonal influenza. It was recommended that we work at home if we could, especially if our work was considered non-essential. We were told to limit gatherings to ten or fewer people and eventually to not "gather" at all.

For many people, embracing these changes was difficult, and some deemed the changes alarmist or unnecessary. Many of us were slow to comply. Many of us got sick and some of us—too many—died. They died alone, isolated from their loved ones. Those loved ones were denied the comfort of funerals and wakes. At the time of writing, people are still dying in great numbers. The comfort of communal grieving is denied to us for the sake of the health of others. I recently lost an old friend to a stroke and, because of the virus, I could not visit her before she passed. I could not offer her treatments for the sequelae of her stroke because the nursing home where she was staying after her hospital stay did not allow visitors. When she was declining, I could not say goodbye. I could not attend a memorial to celebrate her life, because it didn't happen. These restrictions were all necessary to protect everyone but they are painful and stressful restrictions. Like many others, it has been heart-breaking not to be able to spend time with family members that are at high risk. Many of us comply with these restrictions because we cannot imagine the agony and terror of having a loved one hospitalized with this infection.

The infection rate eventually rose so high that we were told that we must, for the safety of all, change our behavior. Non-essential businesses were told to close. People were strongly advised to stay home so that we might "flatten the curve." They closed the schools and parents became teachers overnight. Teachers had to adapt to a new way of reaching their students. Many had to quickly grasp new and challenging technology to try to maintain their business. Others lost their sources of income. Many of us struggled with the loss of social connection. People were beset by worry and anxiety; some even became paranoid and germ-phobic in the extreme. YouTube videos on how to wash your hands, remove disposable gloves and clean your groceries after a trip to the grocery store could be found everywhere on social media. No one could tell if these responses to the pandemic were reasonable because we did not have enough information to really know what was prudent. Many of us were uncomfortable in the choices we had to make. The information about this virus came slowly and, as with all developing science, there were differences of opinion and approach. It was a confusing time.

We were forced into stillness, containment and, for some, an uncomfortable boredom that made the days seem exceptionally long. Some of us lost sleep and some of us began to sleep too much as a way of avoiding the feelings that came with this time of great upheaval, tragedy and loss.

It was a time when an invisible threat was deemed deadly, and to compound that deadliness, we were informed that even people who appeared to be healthy could be spreading the virus. No place and no one was safe. Not to sound Dickensian, but it was a time of great fear and overwhelming worry. We were beset by fear of infection, fear of infecting our loved ones in vulnerable populations, fear of drowning in our own fluids and fear of dying. We also had fears of how this whole situation was being handled. There was great panic and frustration around a lack of available medical supplies and limited access to medical care. Hospitals and health care workers were overwhelmed. On the news, we were hearing daily about the shortage of masks, gowns, testing equipment and ventilators. Once the fears of infection hit their peak, we began to face other fears—economic fears, mental health fears—and many of us were plagued by existential fears of what our futures would be like. What would our new normal look like? These fears gave rise to a plethora of conspiracy theories and conflicting information about how this happened. Who was to blame and what did we need to do to survive this plague? Arguments over whether or not to wear a mask led to violence. It was a time of frustration, resistance and anger. And as if that wasn't enough to deal with, here in the USA we were forced, by blatant police brutality, to once again face the systemic racism that has "plagued" this nation since its beginning. It was a time of fear, and fear is a hallmark of evolutionary stress.

It was also a time of blossoming love and compassion. People were realizing that in a time of great need there was many an opportunity to share and to give. It was a time when we saw amazing acts of courage, kindness and service. People risked their health by going to work every day so that grocery stores would be stocked, hospitals would be cleaned, and buses would be there to take people where they needed to go. People delivered food, medication and toilet paper to those in need. Medical professionals risked their health and the health of their families to treat those affected by the virus. Nurses traveled across the country to support their fellow nurses in the hot spots who were working exhausting hours under impossible conditions. The Black Lives Matters protesters risked their health to stand up for what is right and just.

When I speak of how this pandemic and all that followed was an illustration of the nature of evolutionary stress, I am saying that at a global level we experienced something that, as horrible as it was, gave us the opportunity to re-examine our values and our sense of self.

Evolutionary stress can be any stress that creates enough fear that feels life-threatening or any stressor or trauma that affects our sense of Self. This type of stress can be personal, such as a cancer diagnosis. It can be familial, such as abuse or addiction, or it can be global and systemic, such as misogyny, racism and fascism. It is the type of stress that forces you to adapt or die.

The 8 EV were built for these times and for this type of stress. As the only vessels active *in utero* during gestation, these vessels shape who we are. These are jing vessels and as such they hold the key to our curriculum. They govern how our jing cycles unfold. The Yuan qi aspect of these vessels is manifest in who we are meant to be. They reflect our true temperament, our constitution and Yuan Shen/Original Spirit. They are the source of our authenticity and in them lies the path to self-knowledge, self-love, self-acceptance and the belief that we are an embodied reflection of the Divine and, as such, we are enough.

Just as we forget what it felt like to come into the world, I think we forget that we have these resources available to us. We get so wrapped up in surviving and striving, accumulating and compensating, that we lose sight of who we are. The cost of self-preservation is a distancing from this abundance of pre-natal gifts and a reliance on our post-natal function to get through each day the best that we can. We forget our original nature and we begin to believe the lie that we are what has happened to us. We are deceived, mostly by ourselves, but also by the indoctrination and expectations of others. We fall under the illusion that who we are is defined by our ability to get through challenges, to get over heartbreak, to ignore the judgment of others and to get by in a way that demonstrates our resilience and independence. All excellent life skills, but not who we are. When we are detached from these primary resources, we find our worth in things or in how many people admire or approve of us. We seek validation for our continued existence from outside of ourselves. We lose the ability to validate our own existence. We harbor shame, guilt and self-judgment as critical voices in our heads that beat us down for our efforts to survive. These voices seduce us into believing that they are here to help and that their purpose is to support us to be better, to do better. No critical voice or no shaming voice ever made us better human beings. No amount of self-judgment ever made us feel better about ourselves or solved a problem. Guilt, shame and self-judgment might temporarily alter our behavior, but they won't heal the fear that initiates that behavior. To continue on that path of survival, we may need to create latency for self-preservation. Once we have created the latency, we begin to live a much less authentic life, where resources that should be used for growth are instead used to keep the truth from our hearts. We forget how to love ourselves.

When we create latency at the level of jing, we forget who we are. We experience trauma so deep and so profound that we must create a new and diminished expression of ourselves that can ignore the impact of that trauma. If we cannot process the trauma or release the impact of the trauma, then we must store it in a place that allows us to forget it or pretend it never happened. We create a distance between the experience and our conscious mind. Resources are diverted to support the latency and they get stuck. The lack of circulation further limits our ability to process or release the trauma. Once we create the latency, we stop growing.

The 8 EV can be a very effective way to redirect the impact of trauma and release the latency so that we can get back on track. We can, through these vessels, regain our sovereignty. As these vessels are regulated, we can pursue our curriculum with purpose, and we can relate to ourselves and the world around us in a way that is more in alignment with who we truly are.

If we received any training in these vessels during our education, we were typically taught to look at them from the perspective of master and couple points. Matching them this way puts a master point that opens a sea of resources with a couple point that helps to distribute that resource to a particular area of the body. For example, the master point of the Ren mai is Lu-7. This opens the Sea of Yin and it is coupled with Ki-6 which distributes yin up and down the front of the body. This is a perfectly reasonable way to understand these vessels if you want to address a physical problem. It does not, however, really explain how the evolution of consciousness occurs through this system. It does not explain how jing unfolds over the seven- and eight-year cycles and how resources are allocated for growth. If we want to understand that, we must look at the 8 EV slightly differently.

We begin with the Chong mai. This is the source vessel of the 8 EV. It is undifferentiated yin and yang and it contains within it the potential for life unfolding. It represents unity, oneness, wholeness. But the problem with oneness is that incarnation into a human body for the purpose of living life requires polarity, duality and multiplicity. The Chong mai must then give birth to that polarity in the form of Source Yin and Source Yang. This is the Ren and Du mai. These three vessels represent the resources needed for you to fulfill your curriculum. From here it becomes a matter of how one will distribute and protect those resources.

The Wei Mai distribute those resources over time, adjusting the resources during times of stress and transition. They create a link between the pre-natal resources of the Chong, Ren and Du and the post-natal function of the Zang Fu. The Yang Wei links post-natal yang channels and functions of the Fu organs with the Du mai. The Yin Wei links post-natal yin channels and the functions of the zang organs with the Ren mai. This allows us to maintain a continuity of Self as we age and grow.

The Qiao vessels reach from the heels to the head in a way that allows us to distribute the resources of yin and yang up and down the body to support stance and perspective as we take up space in the world. These vessels support the physical structure for postural alignment and locomotion.

The Dai mai is the final vessel in this unfolding of jing and it serves two purposes. The first is related to its horizontal nature. This circulation around the waist allows the Dai mai to connect and interact with all of the other vessels. This means it can function as a mediator and, in its regulating and harmonizing function, it can provide support for the Chong, Ren and Du. You can think of this function like the lumbar belt that weight-lifters use before they do any heavy lifting. This function creates the stability, centering and integration that allow us to begin to develop appropriate boundaries as we grow.

The second function of the Dai mai is to provide a receptacle for unprocessed trauma that affects our sense of Self. This is how latency is created in the 8 EV. When the Pericardium (Heart Protector) is overwhelmed and cannot protect the Heart from trauma or any experience that threatens consciousness, it pushes that trauma away from the Heart, moving it down into the Dai mai. When the Wei and Qiao vessels are overwhelmed by experience and they cannot maintain distribution of resources, they too will direct the pathogenic nature of the experience down into the Dai mai. The Dai mai's storage nature is designed to preserve life and give us the much-needed time to develop context for the traumas we have experienced and to rally our resources to face that trauma with courage and will. Latency created at this level comes from serious life-altering trauma and it may take many years before we are ready to face the truth and let go.

When we take our first breath in this body and in this world, we activate our post-natal function. Our lungs inflate and we send a message to the rest of the body that it is time to embrace existence. But unlike most of the animal kingdom, we come into the world not fully functioning. We lack a level of independence that is found in most animals after birth. We cannot walk or talk. We cannot hold our heads on top of our spines, so we are unable to maintain an upright position. All babies are vulnerable but human babies even more so. The first cycle of jing is dedicated to building and strengthening our post-natal function for independence. Because our post-natal function is weak in our first seven or eight years, we rely on our pre-natal resources (8 EV) to fund that development. When we have trauma in that first cycle, especially in the first two years, when we are at our most vulnerable, that trauma imprints heavily on the Chong, Ren and Du mai. Early childhood trauma changes who we are. It can take us off the path of our curriculum and put us on a road where the pursuit of survival obstructs a meaningful life. It diverts the resources that are meant to help us fulfill our life's purpose towards maintaining latency for survival. This diversion keeps us living in fear of the next devastating experience. Even when we are not aware, we are anticipating the next crisis. The impact of trauma on the pre-natal gifts we were given by the cosmos and our parents and their parents, changes not only our ability to pursue our destiny but it also impedes the full expression of Self. It negatively impacts self-awareness, self-worth, self-love, self-propulsion and our ability to feel accepted by the world around us. This diversion may, in many of us, lead to a self-destructive search for anything that will take away the hurt feelings and self-loathing. We may turn to alcohol or drugs for comfort. We may turn to food to nourish the black hole that is caused by trauma. We may attract abusive relationships into our lives that support the negative belief that we are unworthy of love.

We are less capable of understanding our part in the trauma of early childhood, as we have not yet reached the age of reason.

This means that whatever we experience in childhood imprints in a very emotional manner. As a result, we may have problems regulating our emotions. We may suffer from anxiety, depression, obsessive thinking or anger management issues. We may learn to manipulate the emotions of others to survive or feel safer. I am saying this because even when we release the latency in the Dai mai and free up resources, if the imprint happens in childhood, we may need to go back and regulate the function of these very important source vessels. We may need to remind people of who they are. We may need to reconnect them with the truth that they are enough and they are worthy of love. We may need to empower them to extend themselves into the world with the understanding that they have the potency needed to act. We do this by restoring healthy function to the Chong, Ren and Du mai.

In the third and fourth cycles of jing, we complete the development of our post-natal function. Our skeletons are fully developed and we are done physically growing. Our hair is as full as it is going to get; we have hit our physical peak. From this point on, it becomes about holding on to resources or, at the very least, using them wisely. Once the infrastructure of post-natal function is built, then we can rely much less on the resources provided by the 8 EV. These resources are typically called upon during the transitions associated with growth and development or at times of evolutionary stress. They are drawn on for fertility and issues associated with the ever-changing terrain of aging. In particular, the 8 EV are deeply connected to the Curious Organs (Extraordinary Fu). These Curious Organs (the uterus, brain, vessels, marrow, bones and the gall bladder) are those in which we can see the ravages of aging. As we age, we lose our fertility, our cognitive function and memory, our cardiovascular health, our bone health and our courage. The 8 EV support the function of the Curious Organs and therefore they are incredibly helpful in managing the process of growing older. Maintaining the health of the Curious Organs can increase longevity and reduce the emotional resistance to the inevitable downhill slide. We can actually enjoy aging and make the most of it.

This does not mean we look forward to getting old and dying. It means that we accept that everyone gets old, everyone dies and gravity always wins. Once we accept that reality, we can actually focus on the here and now, and we can make the most of whatever time we are given. We can learn to enjoy the benefits of aging. As we age, the wisdom that comes from life experience allows us to more easily say, "No, I don't think so." We also seem to care less about what others think and we have refined our values to a point that we know what is truly important. If you are willing to accept the discomforts of aging, what you get in return is freedom.

Once the infrastructure is built and we are no longer physically growing and developing, we begin to rely more on our ability to digest life through post-natal function. We rely on Ying qi as the primary resource for facing the world. We are reserving the pre-natal resources of the 8 EV, especially the Chong, Ren and Du mai, for times of great need.

This is where we can see the effect of trauma on the Wei and Qiao vessels. The Wei vessels "link" pre- and post-natal resources in order to maintain continuity of Self during times of stress or transition. It is a way of saying, "Go now, live your life, use your Ying qi to make decisions, to nourish yourself, to interact with the world around you." "Go and learn things through the function of the Yi/Spleen, but do not forget who you are." When the Wei vessels are impeded by trauma or when they are overwhelmed by life, we lose the pre- and post-natal connection. When we act or feel, it is often out of alignment with who we are. We may act in a way that is self-destructive or we may feel discontented with our lives because we have lost that connection. We also lose our connection to those resources that support the generation of qi and blood. This loss results in qi and blood deficiency, which makes it even more difficult to negotiate transitions well.

The Qiao vessels help us mediate how our feet connect with the ground and how our vision is engaged. When we have structural alignment from the feet up, we can move more effectively in the world. When the Qiao vessels are healthy and in balance, we can direct our vision wherever it will provide the necessary information for living well. We can turn our vision inward for self-illumination or we can focus outward to see what lies ahead. When life's challenges interfere with these vessels, it alters our perspective and stance. This then makes it quite challenging to make our way in the world in a way that accurately reflects who we are.

If the Chong mai is the Alpha, then the Dai mai is the Omega. It represents the culmination of the unfolding of jing. The Dai mai has two basic functions, one that is pre-natal in nature and one that is post-natal. The pre-natal nature of the Dai mai has to do with its horizontal pathway. As the only horizontal channel in the body, its pathway comes in direct contact with other vertical pathways. This is where we see the regulating, integrating and harmonizing functions of the Dai mai. Once again, you can think of this path as a lumbar support belt. It provides a consolidating force that holds everything together in the lower jiao. This pathway creates a loop around the waist that runs from Du-4 in the back, to GB-26 on the flank and Ren-8 in the front of the body. Additional points along this pathway also include UB-23, UB-52, Sp-15, St-25 and Ki-16. This consolidating force provides an avenue for communication between the Chong, Du and Ren, which is essential for the creation of healthy boundaries in childhood. If a child experiences trauma during the development of these boundaries, then the ability to consolidate the Dai mai and its relationship between the Chong, Du and Ren will be impaired, and patients will be left feeling unsupported in life.

The post-natal nature of the Dai mai provides a receptacle for unprocessed traumas, challenges and beliefs that threaten to destroy a patient's sense of Self or activate their need for survival. So often experiences that initiate the creation of latency in the Dai mai are experiences that feel life-threatening or those that make you feel as if you want to die. One does not stuff something down into the Dai mai because it is a little uncomfortable. One uses the Dai mai as a storage basin to avoid or forget things that are so awful that we don't think we can live with them. The pathway for this function is slightly different. The back of the girdle is the same—Du-4, UB-23 and UB-52—but the front includes Lv-13, GB-26, GB-27 and GB-28. When you connect the dots on these points, you have something that resembles a bucket more than a belt.

When latency is created in the Dai mai, stagnation occurs, and dampness is generated to secure the pathogen in the nether regions of the body. This accounts for the typical physical manifestations of Dai mai pathology that include vaginal discharge, diarrhea, weight gain around the middle and thighs, and difficulty rotating the waist. This dampness creates further stagnation which very effectively blocks the Heart and Kidney (Shen and Zhi) axis. This divides the body into two halves. The Heart is protected from the unprocessed trauma, which is deposited in the lower jiao and covered by pathogenic fluids. We have survived but we are cut off from our source. Many types of traumatic experiences can trigger the drive to create latency in the Dai mai for survival purposes, but most of those experiences reflect a violation of boundaries.

When it comes to releasing the Dai mai, you must be careful that you do not further traumatize the patient. This act of self-preservation is the deepest form of distancing you can create. Freeing up the Dai mai is essential in order to restore the Heart and Kidney axis, but one must do it carefully with respect. The patient created the latency because they felt violated, so we must not do anything that further violates the patient's trust. It is most important that we make sure that the patient has enough resources to effectively and comfortably release. Are they robust enough? Is their constitution strong enough? Are they able to rest or have the down time needed to process the release? Do they have family and social support? Will they need therapeutic support?

If you cannot be sure they have the necessary support and they still want to clear the Dai mai, then it is advisable to use the pre-natal pathway and consolidate the Dai mai first. In fact, when in doubt, consolidate. Although consolidating might seem like the opposite direction of draining, it is often useful to consolidate the primary resources of the Chong, Du and Ren mai through the pre-natal pathway of the Dai mai. In this way, the patient has enough support to choose to release the latency on their own. These patients tend to present with dampness associated with Spleen qi deficiency or Spleen qi sinking. Their pattern tends to be deficient and cold. Suppressed emotions in these patients are often associated with fear and shame. Consolidating would be done by inserting the master point GB-41 and then choosing from the following points: Du-4, UB-23, UB-52, GB-26, Sp-15, St-25, Ki-16 or Ren-8. It is not necessary to add SJ-5 (couple point) to this treatment. The focus is on cinching the belt, not venting the pathogen.

If the patient is robust enough and they have adequate support, then you can drain the Dai mai. These patients typically present with a level of toxicity or damp-heat in their symptoms. Their pathology is clearly excess in nature. They are often suffering from Liver fire, Gall Bladder damp-heat or damp-heat in the lower jiao. Suppressed emotions are most often linked to frustration, bitterness, resentment and rage. Draining the Dai mai would still begin with the master point GB-41 and then you would choose from the points on the post-natal pathway. Those include: Lv-13, GB-26, GB-27, GB-28. Add the couple point SJ-5 to increase the venting function and to facilitate heat-clearing.

Once the Dai mai is cleared, you may need to regulate the function of the other 8 EV. I have talked at great length about the functions of each of the vessels in my previous book (Farrell 2016) and I do not want to repeat myself. I believe it will suffice to give you a sort of encapsulated essence of each of these vessels. This will, I hope, allow you to see where pathology still exists in the 8 EV after clearing the Dai mai. You may then be able to go back and regulate the imbalances that were overwhelmed enough to create the need for latency in the first place. So what follows is a limited or condensed view of the primary psycho-emotional functions of each vessel and the hallmark existential crises associated with each.

CHONG MAI

This is the blueprint for life. It is pure potential and the vehicle for genetic transmission. This channel links pre- and post-natal function by connecting the Kidney to the Stomach and Spleen along its pathway. It provides pre-natal resources for the creation of post-natal substances through digestion. The hallmark crisis in the Chong is existential indeed. When there is pathology, we have either forgotten who we are or we are burdened by intergenerational trauma or cultural expectations. This vessel takes us back to the source and allows us to decide if the baggage we are carrying is ours, or if the baggage comes from our ancestors. It may also help us to free ourselves from the weight of this baggage so that we do not pass it down to the next generation.

REN MAI

Archetypally, this vessel represents the feminine (yin), especially the mother. It gifts us with the ability to conceive of something, gestate it, labor over it, give it birth, nurture it and then, with unconditional love, let it go. This vessel is about facilitating yin. When there is pathology in this vessel, we see difficulty in healthy bonding and lack of self-love or self-care, especially when it revolves around nourishment. This vessel also has a very strong impact on the directed flow of qi. Three of the most powerful qi-regulating points on the body can be found on the Ren (Ren-17, Ren-12 and Ren-6). We often see patients with Ren mai pathology suffering from qi stagnation disorders such as pre-menstrual syndrome, bloating and anxiety. This form of qi stagnation, from a Ren mai perspective, is a tension that might be described as over-containment. These patients have lost the softening function of yin and they are wrapped too tightly, like a mother who just cannot let go.

DU MAI

Archetypally, this vessel represents the masculine, especially the father or figures of authority. This vessel gives us potency, curiosity and motive force to explore the world. It gives us the strength to stand upright and separate from our mothers. When there is a weakness in the Du, we see a loss of motive force, apathy, difficulty individuating, a lack of courage or someone who is easily discouraged. In some people, pathology in the Du mai presents as an excess of yang and patients will have anger management issues. They may be aggressively independent or independent too early in life.

YIN WEI

This vessel links the Ren mai to the post-natal yin channels, organs and functions. It provides continuity of Self through the major transitions in life. It helps us to manage the feelings associated with changes in our bodies during the aging process. It manages the emotions of rites and passages such as puberty and menopause. The Yin Wei helps us to internalize experience. When there is pathology, it is usually marked by feelings of discontent. We are unsatisfied occupying our bodies and our lives. We are prone to fantasy thinking that makes it challenging to stay in the moment and embrace reality. This lack of ability to link results in heartbreak. The Yin Wei is said to treat the nine kinds of Heart pain.

YANG WEI

This vessel links the Du mai to the post-natal yang channels, organs and functions. It manages action or behavior during the aging process. It allows us to divert resources for movement that are appropriate to the time. It helps us to manage right-action. This vessel has a strong affinity with the nature of Shao Yang and it has a strong venting function. Pathology usually involves some sort of self-sabotage and might include passive-aggressive behavior, futile or wasteful action or action that is inconsistent with age. Most patients with Yang Wei pathology report a "stuckness" in their lives.

YIN QIAO

The Yin Qiao is about alignment and insight. It governs structural alignment from the arch of the foot up to the head. It turns the vision inward for self-illumination. When there is pathology here, it affects alignment and causes problems with the deep stabilizing muscles of the body, including the sphincter muscles. It is very common to see yin pathogens (cold, damp and blood) get stuck in the abdomen. We might see all sorts of lumpy-bumpy things that are very commonly associated with gynecological and obstetric disorders. When the vision is affected, patients have trouble seeing themselves realistically. They may have an unhealthy body image or may even feel possessed. Gu syndrome is a condition that is frequently associated with Yin Qiao patterns. It affects not only the digestive function but also neurological function. This possession, which obstructs the abdomen and also cognition, makes it difficult for patients to trust.

YANG QIAO

Locomotion and the ability to see what is up ahead are the primary functions of the Yang Qiao. This is the ability to put one foot in front of the other and move forward. Pathology manifests as obstruction in the head, tunnel vision, difficulty with locomotion and musculo-skeletal pain. The Yang Qiao is very Tai Yang in nature and, as a result, it has the ability to set the threshold of response to external stimuli. It determines how much information gets in and what our reflexive response to that information will be. As the system becomes overwhelmed, we might see things like headaches, especially sinus-related headaches. This is a reflection of the Yang Qiao's ability to use the fluids of Tai Yang (Urinary Bladder) to create a veil that reduces input. We might also see the Wei qi response become overreactive to external stimuli. It is common, for instance, to see this in patients with PTSD.

DAI MAI

The Dai mai regulates, integrates and harmonizes the channel system. It is essential to the development of healthy boundaries. It provides a receptacle for the suppression of unprocessed trauma for survival purposes. Pathology in this channel usually involves Shadow work—bringing into the light that which we have hidden from ourselves and letting it go. As mentioned earlier, violation of boundaries is usually a factor in pathology.

Here are some key points that are important if you are doing 8 EV treatments:

- The master point is the first point inserted. Think of it as the key that unlocks the door. There are techniques you can use to access Yuan qi but until you learn them, you can use your intent. It is usually done unilaterally. It only takes one key to unlock the door.

- Location for the master points is slightly different. Needle the yin channel master points in the biggest dip or crevice. Needle the yang channel master points where the skin and fascia bundle the most. This is most obvious in the master points for the Qiao vessels. Ki-6 is found in the large depression closer to the bottom of the foot than the anatomical location. UB-62 is needled underneath the tendons that bunch below the lateral malleolus. The needle may be inserted posterior to the tendons, allowing the needle to pass under the tendons.

- The couple point may be useful but is not always necessary. If you have a patient who needs an 8 EV treatment, they are not processing well. Each channel or needle you include is a piece of information that will need to be processed. Less is more. Sometimes the couple point adds to the intent of the treatment. For instance, it is not necessary to add Pc-6 to a Chong mai treatment but it may be helpful to open the chest and diaphragm.

- Add points on the pathway of the chosen vessel to reinforce your intent. Do less and choose wisely. Remember that the point is less important than the channel. The channel does the heavy lifting; the individual points refine the details. If you are doing a Du mai treatment, it is not necessary to do a ton of Du points to get the point across. Using two points will do the job; use three if you are not doing any other points.

- One should avoid any points that are not in or connected to the Yuan level. These points would be considered a distraction. They may dilute, weaken or confuse the intent of the treatment. In effect, additional points that are not connected to the Yuan level may ruin the efficacy of the treatment.

- If you feel the overwhelming need to add a point or two that are not on the pathway of the vessel you choose, pick from the following point classifications that are associated with Yuan qi: He-sea, front-mu, back-shu, Influential points, San Jiao points, Kidney points, upper and lower meeting points of the Divergent channels and Luo points.

- Needles should be retained for 40 minutes from the time the first needle (master point) is inserted.

- Treatments are usually done once a week, then spaced further apart when things start to move or change. Activating these powerful pre-natal resources is instantaneous, but using the information they provide takes time. The patient must process that information and establish new patterns of behavior and awareness. Some people take longer to process than others and some messages are so powerful they require more time to unfold.

- One course of treatment is considered to be three months (108 days). This is the length of time it takes to change or mobilize jing. This is something we see in fertility treatments. It takes three months to change sperm parameters and three months to regulate the menstrual cycle. Change may occur after the first treatment but stabilizing that change may take a little time.

KEYS TO SELF-HELP FOR THE 8 EV

You may refer to the suggestions I gave for Yuan qi and the Divergents: breathe, find stillness and engage the Observer. These activities will help you to access the depths of the 8 EV, too.

I seldom recommend that practitioners treat themselves. It is an important thing to surrender and allow others to objectively and compassionately care for us. However, the 8 EV are vessels of destiny and who better to take charge of your destiny than you? If you do not want to needle yourself, then you can use essential oils to activate the points. You can also use magnets, tacks, seeds and lasers, but I usually recommend the essential oils because they are plant jing. I like the resonance. Jeffrey Yuen offered in one class the following oils for each of the 8 EV. Choose one and apply it sparingly with a toothpick or a guide tube.

Table 9.1 Essential oils for use with the 8 EV

Chong mai	Sage, Fennel, Myrrh, Frankincense
Ren mai	Ginger, Pine, Juniper, Cypress
Du mai	Rosemary or Fennel
Dai mai	Gentiana, Lavender, German (Blue) Chamomile
Yin Wei	Sage, Clary Sage, Angelica, Sandalwood
Yang Wei	Petitgrain, Orange, Lemon, Grapefruit, Bergamot, Neroli
Yin Qiao	Sweet Marjoram or Thyme
Yang Qiao	Lavender, Roman (Yellow) Chamomile, Spearmint, Peppermint

Many of the symptoms of 8 EV pathology overlap and it may be difficult to know exactly where to begin. If you cannot decide, Jeffrey Yuen recommends you start at the beginning (Chong mai) or the end (Dai mai). Almost everyone has pathology in either or both of those. Do the treatment with as much intent as you can muster up and then engage the Observer and watch what happens. These vessels can help you to live life at the mythic level. They help you to embrace the Hero's Journey. They support you in expressing yourself in the most powerfully authentic manner possible. Be who you are and live your life boldly, with courage, compassion and empathy. These are qualities that can be nourished through the 8 EV.

A DAI MAI CASE STUDY

It would be easy at this point to present to you a Dai mai case study filled with self-preservation arising from sexual abuse and the violation of boundaries. I have seen so many patients who are suffering the impact of early childhood violation. You can no doubt recognize that type of severe trauma and its impact on the Dai mai. The case I have chosen for you is more subtle and not so easily seen.

The patient is a male, in his late 50s, who reported having "feelings of low energy," "feeling ill with no symptoms" and having episodes of dread when he was certain that he "was going to die." These feelings started a couple of months before his first visit. He was cleared after examination by an MD. There was no apparent cause for the feelings or for the extreme but intermittent fatigue. He had some family stress and loss in the last couple of years, which he felt he was handling well. He is happily married to his childhood sweetheart and he has two adult children. His medical history included surgery for kidney stones, psoriasis (mild and not easily visible) and tension in the mid-back and diaphragm that sometimes affected his breathing. In general, he has a robust constitution, sturdy build and a fitness level that is confirmed by reports of regular mountain biking. His demeanor is gregarious and he is quick to laugh and an excellent story-teller. In the year prior to his first visit, he had a terrible accident while riding his bicycle on a challenging trail. He broke his collar bone and four ribs, and although he did not lose consciousness, he definitely feared for his life. I felt pretty sure that I was going to be dealing with the Yang Qiao as the musculo-skeletal injury and fall triggered a Wei qi response that could indeed be the source of his uncomfortable feelings and fatigue. I was a little surprised that his pulse reflected Dai mai pathology (large and more forceful in the middle position, Liver and Spleen). This was further confirmed by a tongue that was dusky-red with a yellow greasy coat. The only Dai mai symptom he claimed to have was a sense of fullness in the lower abdomen. We talked about the accident and I began to see how braced he was when he spoke about it.

The first two treatments were Dai mai and Yin Wei treatments.

Ten needles were used in the following order:

GB-41: Open the Dai mai.

Pc-6: Open the Yin Wei, support release of the diaphragm and relaxation of the Pericardium loop. I normally do not add an additional vessel to the first treatment. I prefer to keep things as simple as possible on the first visit. I could not shake the idea that the "bracing" he was experiencing was a form of anxiety.

Even though he did not feel anxious, there was something anticipatory in his demeanor.

Sp-8: Di Ji/Earth mechanism, xi-cleft point to wake the Spleen and remove dampness obstructing the Dai mai. This point is not on the pathway of either the Dai mai or the Yin Wei but its damp-reducing function and its ability to support transformation and transportation is very consistent with both the Dai mai and Yin Wei.

GB-26: Dai mai, most lateral point on both the pre-natal and post-natal Dai.

Lv-14: Yin Wei point. Qi Men/Cycle Gate, last point on the Liver channel, end of the Ying qi cycle. This is about endings creating the possibility of new beginnings.

Lu-2 threaded to Lu-1: Front-mu point of the Lungs and first point on the Ying qi cycle. This is about starting anew. When we are asking patients to start over after a trauma it may be important to find a way to initiate new beginnings in the flow of qi. The combination of Lv-14 and Lu-1 does this. Using the front-mu point of the Lung also supports the Po's ability to let go of the body memory of the accident that is stuck in the sinews.

This treatment produced excellent results for about three days. He was able to easily ride his bike and he had no more feelings of dread. The symptoms returned after a trail ride in which he felt he overdid it and set himself back. I did not see it that way. I think he is passionate about trail-riding. It is an essential part of how he takes care of himself. I think what happened is the ride got a little dangerous or challenging and this triggered the fear of the accident and he then braced the Pericardium loop and stuffed the fear down once again. Stuffing down the fear is essential if he is to continue pursuing his passion. This blocked the Dai mai and the feelings came back. The good news was that when they returned, they were not as bad as the feelings of dread that first brought him to me. We repeated the treatment with two small changes. Instead of Sp-8, I used Ki-9. Ki-9/Zhu Bin is the xi-cleft point of the Yin Wei. This point helps us take up residence in our lives in the here and now. I also used GB-21 instead of Lu-2 threaded to Lu-1. Once the new beginning was initiated, I felt it was more important to help him let go of the burden he was carrying. GB-21 is sometimes known as the "Atlas" point, named after Atlas, the son of a Titan, who was condemned to hold the weight of the Heavens for eternity. Over time, it has come to mean one that carries the weight of the world on his shoulders; but it is not the world Atlas was condemned to carry—it was the weight of the Cosmos. He was condemned for his part in the war against the gods of Olympus. He was found guilty and punished for his part in going against the gods. Sometimes when we risk ourselves and fail, we are beset by guilt and that is a heavy burden. My intent with using GB-21 was to help this patient let go of the guilt he might feel for risking himself to pursue his passion. Accidents happen. After that treatment, he was feeling significantly better and he had better awareness of how to take care of himself on his rides.

After the first two treatments, his tongue was much less red and the coat was thinner. The feelings of extreme fatigue and dread were down to a manageable 3/10. He was riding regularly and the fatigue he experienced after a ride was normal for the exertion. His pulse changed. It was no longer a Dai mai pulse and his tongue coat was almost cleared ("almost" being the operative word here, stay tuned). He had just a little patch of greasiness between the areas associated with the middle and lower jiao. He was now presenting with a pulse that I recognize as being consistent with the Yang Qiao. This is what I expected to treat the first time I met with him, so it made sense to me that it was time to address the musculo-skeletal part of the trauma.

Ah hubris, thy name is Yvonne. I'll admit here that I am a Fire type. I like to get to the point quickly. I often move faster than is prudent. I am just so excited by the fact that things are happening. I refer you to recommendation number 1 in Chapter 4: **The patient takes the lead** *and the practitioner brakes*. One of my biases is I like to go fast; not coincidentally, so does this patient.

The Yang Qiao treatment was as follows:

UB-62: Master point of the Yang Qiao, left side.

UB-59: Xi-cleft point of the Yang Qiao, also done on the left.

UB-23: Back-shu point of the Kidneys but also on the posterior portion of the Dai mai.

Du-9: For emotional constraint, opens the diaphragm for the tension in the chest.

UB-43: Outer-shu point of the Pericardium. The Pericardium's job is to protect the Heart by bearing the unbearable. When it can no longer do that, it stuffs the pathogen down into the Dai mai.

SI-10: To address the bracing of Tai Yang in the region of the shoulder and upper back.

GB-21: To support the release of Shao Yang for flexibility in the face of change. Helps the patient adapt and opens Shao Yang for an expanded perspective.

Du-16: For the tightness in the neck but also to access the brain to address the Curious Organ's part in holding on to the trauma.

Such a good treatment, I thought. Let's help the patient to free the body and mind so that they can move forward and pursue their passion without anticipatory fear. I had a plan and you know what they say about God and plans.

The patient had a pretty awful week after this treatment. He was unable to ride at all. He felt so bad that he didn't want to do anything. Lucky for me, the feeling that he was dying did not return but he basically felt terrible for a week. He was also more aware of the chest restriction. His pulse was a diaphragm pulse, felt most strongly between the index and ring fingers. The constriction in the chest was most evident in the pulse. It became very obvious after this treatment that the Dai mai pathology had not completely resolved, and if I was going to try to release the body memory, I probably should have done some sinew work, such as gua sha or cupping, on the mid-back. I went back to the Yin Wei and Dai mai in an attempt to reclaim the forward progress we made in the first two treatments.

Pc-6: Master point of the Yin Wei. I made this the first point because of the constriction in the chest. As master point of the Yin Wei, it opens the chest and diaphragm and helps the patient to internalize experience.

GB-41: Master point of the Dai mai. For the unresolved trauma.

Ki-9: Xi-cleft point of Yin Wei. Unblocks the Yin Wei and helps patients take up residence in their own lives.

Sp-15: Point on the Yin Wei that supports transformation and transportation. It is also a point on the pre-natal (consolidating) Dai mai.

Lv-14: Front-mu point of Liver. Qi Men/Cycle Gate, endings and beginnings, starting over. This point also opens the diaphragm for emotional constraint.

Ren-15: Luo point of the Ren mai and upper point of the Bao Mai. To restore the connection between the Pericardium and Dai mai.

Lu-2 to Lu-1: As before, new beginnings and support of the Po.

After this treatment, the patient had a good week. He had one day when he was tired but not bad. We still have not resolved this sense of tension in the chest. He is quite sure it is not associated with shortness of breath as he can experience it and still take a deep breath and ride his bike. We have begun to speak about his long history of worrying. He says he has worried since he was a child and most people are not aware of that because he has learned over time to compensate, as we all do, for that reaction to stress. Now the goal is to see if we can find where the latency has been created in order to compensate for this worry. His energy is good. His rides are challenging and tiring but not exhausting. He has begun doing some guided meditations with his wife as a way of reducing stress and becoming more body-aware. He still has some very slight greasy patches on his tongue, which is a reminder that he is still holding on to some old patterns or beliefs that are stuck in the Dai mai, but he is functioning at a much higher level in terms of quality of life in the six weeks of treatment. It is likely, at this point, that we will begin to move his treatments a little further apart to see if he can sustain the changes created by these treatments.

For me, the magic of the 8 EV treatments is that they hold within them everything you need to be the person you are meant to be. Releasing the Dai mai and regulating all of the other vessels gives us the opportunity to feel the wholeness that is always there. The 8 EV bring us back into the consciousness that validates our existence. If we have alignment in these vessels, life is easier because we are more conscious. When we are more aware, we can more readily choose when survival is essential and when it is important to put our resources towards thriving. We can understand that the creation of latency for survival is a temporary function, not a long-term approach to living that eventually leads to those chronic degenerative diseases that rob us of quality of life. If we remember that the resources are there, then we can, through the evolution of our consciousness, gain access to them and thrive.

WHY CHOOSE AN 8 EV TREATMENT?

These are broad-band vessels that cover all levels of qi. The first ancestry (Chong, Du and Ren) are the pre-natal seas that are repositories of vital resources. The Chong is the Sea of Yuan qi and the Sea of Blood which gives us access to Ying and Yuan qi. The Du mai is the Sea of Yang, which allows us to influence Wei and Yuan qi. The Ren mai is the Sea of Yin, and Ying qi travels in the blood which is a yin substance. Through these vessels, we can support the post-natal channels and we can regulate their function.

The question then becomes: Why would we not always do an 8 EV treatment? The answer to that is these are jing vessels and as such they should be reserved for times of great need. They are archetypal in nature and we call on them when a particular problem seems to be a repeated theme in the patient's life. These vessels provide the precious resources for life's epic journey. Each of the vessels has a nature that can be seen in the recurring themes of a life.

The Chong mai and its Sea of Blood link us to our past. We call our family history a bloodline. The themes associated with this have to do with lineage, intergenerational trauma and cultural or familial expectation. The Sea of Yuan qi aspect of the Chong mai has to do with authenticity. The themes are typically about the existential crisis that occurs when we forget who we are.

The Du mai is the Sea of Yang. Themes here center around not having enough yang (loss of potency) for independence, individuation and the initiation of movement. We might also see yang run amok. Too much yang means themes revolve around a lack of self-control.

The Ren mai is the Sea of Yin. The themes that emerge when the Ren mai is out of balance have to do with the ability to connect and contain. We see issues around unhealthy bonding or the capacity to contain or hold on to something. We may see patients who cannot love themselves or care for themselves in a way that sustains or nourishes.

The Yin Wei links pre- and post-natal yin in a way that is supposed to maintain continuity of self through life's transitions. The theme is typically centered around a sense of discontent. These patients would sell their souls to be anyone else. They have great difficulty in taking up residence in their own lives.

The Yang Wei links pre- and post-natal yang in a way that is supposed to support healthy action appropriate to aging. Themes around this vessel have to do with an inability to pursue right-action. We see a history of action or behavior that is counter-productive.

The Yin Qiao is about internal alignment. Themes here reflect an inability to achieve states of insight or self-illumination that keep us aligned with our purpose or the truth of who we are.

The Yang Qiao is about locomotion. Themes reflect how we make our way in the world.

The Dai mai and its two aspects have to do with integration, mediation, harmony and the need to create latency for survival. Themes that reflect Dai mai pathology include feeling unsupported, violation of boundaries, guilt, shame and betrayal.

Even though these vessels have a broad impact on the whole meridian system, we must still take care when we decide to do an 8 EV treatment. It may be true, for instance, that you can treat an acute exterior cold attack with the Yang Qiao. As I have said in class many times, even though you can, it is a little like shooting a fly with a cannon. It will do the job but it is a terrible waste of resources. We save the 8 EV for the big stuff.

The only thing I have to add to that is this: At the time of writing this chapter, all hell is breaking loose in the USA and the world. The big stuff is happening and people are fighting valiantly for their lives. Please do not be afraid to support your patients at the level of jing. The evolution of humanity may depend on it.

CONCLUSION

Redundancy, Self-Awareness and the Miracle of Survival

To be whole does not mean we are perfect. Wholeness is not about being free of flaws or defects. Our wholeness includes these flaws and defects. What makes us whole is self-acceptance and self-awareness. This is not a static state of beingness. It is not a point of arrival. It is a heroic journey, a process. It is alchemical and requires effort and dedication. In medieval times, the practice of alchemy was concerned with turning base metals into gold. This is the practice of turning something ordinary into something special or extraordinary. It is about the creation of something sacred or divine out of something profane. This is a sort of magical transformation, and when we accomplish it, we often cannot explain how it happened. A sculptor who takes an ordinary lump of marble and turns it into an ethereal representation of the physical form does not make the ethereal form. It already exists in the marble. He just discovers or uncovers it, if you will, by taking away that which is not the wholeness of the resulting form. We are already whole. We just need to let go of the baggage that makes it impossible to see the nature of our beingness.

The spiritual aspect of alchemy is the effort we make to free ourselves from our fears, our self-judgment, our limiting beliefs about who we are and what we are able to accomplish. This is about coming to a state of self-acceptance that acknowledges our right to exist as an emanation of the Divine. This lifetime process is a never-ending journey. To those who think the effort is too great or the journey too long, I would say that each step we take on this journey returns to us a piece of ourselves. No step, no matter how small, is a waste of time or effort because each step makes us more of who we are. Every effort we make towards consciousness will make life better.

When we are confronted with threat, we have the ability to respond to that threat in numerous ways. We can survive unimaginable challenges that assault us at the levels of Wei, Ying and Yuan qi. If the challenge comes from the outside, our Wei qi and sinews will rally in an effort to protect us from the threat. If they cannot manage the threat by bracing against it or expelling it, then the threat moves inward. You might think that the work of the sinews is over with at this point, but no. The sinews and Wei qi will learn from that experience and they will add that information to their reflexive response. A failed Wei qi response trains the Wei qi to become more vigilant, awaiting the next threat. This changes how we hold ourselves so that we can be better prepared for the next challenge. The Wei qi begins to see trouble everywhere and the message it sends to the sinews is that a defensive posture is needed in order to survive. This "brace for impact" response is learned, so it can be unlearned. Staying tense and alert requires a tremendous amount of effort; it is exhausting and rarely necessary. This is energy that could be used for healthy interaction in the world. It is energy that could be used for exploration. This energy could feed our curiosity about the world around us. If our demeanor is relaxed or, at the very least, less defensive, then our body language will convey openness and availability. This more relaxed state is seen and felt by others and it changes how people respond to us.

When the threat is in the interior, then we can respond by making an effort to digest the experience and create some context for it, so we might learn and grow. We can put our attention on the experience during this digestive process, separating what is useful from what is harmful. We can eliminate the harmful information and we can hold on to that which is nourishing and will help us grow. When our digestion is weak or overwhelmed, our Primary channels will engage the Luo-collaterals and they will create latency by taking the threat and moving it into the peripheral circulation, so that the organs are not directly affected. This latency is an active process that requires maintenance. While we are engaged in this process, we are less able to interact with others. Relationships become stressed. We have less patience or tolerance for the needs and differences of others. We do not have the energy for self-reflection and we will find it difficult to learn and grow in relationship. Humans are communal by nature. We need each other and we need connection. Isolation is not good for us. If we cannot nourish ourselves, we cannot nourish an intimate or authentic relationship with others.

When we experience life-altering events that push the Pericardium beyond what is bearable, we can still survive. At the level of Yuan qi, survival means suppressing the pain and moving it away from our conscious awareness. As we have seen, we can do this through the Divergent channels by shunting the pathogen into the joints. The chronic, degenerative pain that results from this suppression is a distraction from the emotional devastation of the trauma. Its slow progression protects organ function and gives us time to gather our resources. The cost of doing this is a disruption of the relationship between Wei qi and Yuan qi. It compromises authentic expression and changes how others perceive us.

We can also address trauma at the level of Yuan qi by dumping it into the Dai mai. This is a way of moving the trauma so deep into the constitution that we need to become less of who we are in order to keep it there. To maintain latency in the Dai mai, we need to forget. We forget the experience but, in the forgetting, we are also distanced from parts of ourselves. To come out of this state of suppression, we must be willing to do the work of the Shadow.

We need to be willing to engage our courage and will to face our fears by shining a light in the dark places. We must be willing to suspend our self-judgment because what often emerges when we free up the Dai mai is the guilt, shame, rage, victimization and martyrdom we have tried to avoid. This process requires a stout heart and a tremendous amount of compassion. If we can manage this a little at a time, each step gets us closer to the part of us that was never injured by the trauma. We regain the place in ourselves where we can see our wholeness.

In engineering, redundancy is a specific system design which is about creating back-ups in case of failure. This usually has a negative connotation because it is generally thought that duplicating components is wasteful or perhaps a result of bad planning. You can think of it as a way of trying to cover your ass, just in case you didn't think of a way of dealing with every possible problem. I think redundancy is something to be celebrated in humanity. Existence is messy and failure is a huge part of the human condition. I think we are very lucky to have so much redundancy built into the system to make sure we have every possible chance at survival. If our Wei qi fails, our Luo-collaterals step in. If the Luos are unable to handle the problem, then the Primary channels send it into the Divergents. If we cannot address the issue through the post-natal channels, then we have the 8 EV and their pre-natal resources which can be used to manage the problem. That is a lot of system support for survival. The longer we live, the more opportunity we have to refine ourselves, to turn ourselves into gold or, as the Taoists might say, to become Jade.

Chinese Medicine has given us the theories of yin and yang and the Five Elements as a way of understanding the mysteries of the Cosmos, the nature of the world around us and what it means to be human. We humans are a reflection of Nature and the Universe. We are apportioned by the Heavens a specific balance between yin and yang and a unique distribution of the Five Elements that make up our constitution. These resources were gifted to us so that we may fulfill our purpose for being here. They support the pursuit of our destiny. We are meant for something. We are here for a reason.

In order to fulfill that curriculum, we have to rely on acts of self-preservation to keep us alive long enough to understand and pursue our purpose. The more awareness we have about the nature of these acts of self-preservation, the more quickly we can mitigate the costs of such acts. This can return to us the resources necessary for a life of meaning. In earlier chapters (5–9), I mention some self-help activities you can engage in to increase the awareness of the state of each system and resolve the latency or resistance.

If you are ready or if you are brave, I would add the following: Listen to the whispers of your heart. Unchecked desire may lead to obsession but desire ignored is even more devastating.

Every step you take towards consciousness is a triumphant act that gives value to all acts of self-preservation. Becoming more aware is a way to honor what it took to get you to this point in time. You are an emanation of the Universe in its entirety. This means everything you did to get to this moment was essential. The Heavens want you to be fully human. Your divine purpose is, in part, the journey towards remembering and accepting yourself fully. Even when you are deeply challenged by the events in the world today, you can know, in your heart, that anything you do to increase your awareness can influence the state of the world around you. The journey of a lifetime begins with a single step. There is no need to do all of the recommendations, every day. Pick one thing and focus your attention on it.

You are at your best when you can access your humanity. When that sounds complicated or impossible to achieve, remember that being who you are is as easy as breathing. You have spent your life working so hard to be someone you are not. You have worn so many masks and carried so much baggage that you are wilting under the weight of it all. Now it is time to surrender, breathe in, exhale and let it go.

You have experienced pain, loss and seemingly insurmountable suffering. So much suffering that you have had to lose yourself to survive it. I want you to know that, even in your darkest hours, what is essentially you is never lost. Who you are is, and always will be, available to you. The essence of who you are is not injured by traumatic experiences or the acts of self-preservation that have helped you to survive.

Take up residence in your life with purpose and determination and then share that truth with the world. Let the truth of who you are express itself in the world as an act of kindness. Let it come forth as a deeply held empathy for those who are near broken with the weight of the judgment of others. Let who you are manifest as a prayer of compassion for those who are so possessed by hatred that they do not recognize their own self-loathing. Express yourself through righteous action that says, "I see your pain but I cannot allow the perpetuation of that pain as an act of violence to go unchallenged." Take a stand, draw a line and then hold it, peacefully, with everything that you are. If you want to share your heart, feed someone, cook for them, feed them love, feed them laughter. Create, draw, write, sculpt, paint, grow flowers for the bees or veggies for your family and friends. Each of these acts is heroic and even if you only do one of them, one time, you will become more human.

You were built for this and for these times. You need never doubt your capacity. On the day that the seed of your existence was planted, you were already given everything you need to be who you are and to pursue your destiny. Do one thing, any thing that moves you in the direction of consciousness, and your life will be better, the world will be better.

Today my one thing is to love, fully, boldly, unabashedly, with everything I am. I share that love with you. You are a miracle, my beloved, and your value to the world and these times cannot be measured.

References

Farrell, Y.R. (2016) *Psycho-Emotional Pain and the Eight Extraordinary Vessels.* London: Singing Dragon.

Herman, A. (2014) *meant to wake up feeling.* New York, NY: great weather for MEDIA, LLC.

Jung, C.G. (1975) *The Collected Works of C. G. Jung, Volume 8: Structures & Dynamics of the Psyche.* RFC Hull (trans.) Princeton, NJ: Princeton University Press.

Lothian, J.A. (2004) "Do not disturb: The importance of privacy in labor." *Journal of Perinatal Education 13,* 3, 4–6.

Lu, H.C. (trans.) (2004) *A Complete Translation of the Nei-Jing and Nan-Jing: The Yellow Emperor's Classic of Internal Medicine and the Difficult Classic.* Vancouver, BC: International College of Traditional Chinese Medicine.

Quinn, B. and Moreland, E. (2008) "Gu Syndrome: An in-depth interview with Heiner Fruehauf." Accessed on October 2, 2020 at https://classicalchinesemedicine.org/gu-syndrome-in-depth-interview-with-heiner-fruehauf.

Suggested Reading

Campbell, J. and Moyers, B. (1991) *The Power of Myth*. New York, NY: Anchor Books.

Cecil-Sterman, A. (2012) *Advanced Acupuncture: A Clinical Manual*. New York, NY: Classical Wellness Press.

Chödrön, P. (1997) *When Things Fall Apart: Heart Advice for Difficult Times*. Boston, MA: Shambala Publications.

Farrell, Y.R. (2016) *Psycho-Emotional Pain and the Eight Extraordinary Vessels*. London: Singing Dragon.

Flaws, B. (trans.) (2004) *Li Dong Yuan's Treatise on the Spleen and Stomach: A Translation of the Pi Wei Lun*. Portland, OR: Blue Poppy Press.

Lipton, B.H. (2005) *The Biology of Belief: Unleashing the Power of Consciousness, Matter and Miracles*. London: Hay House.

Maté, G. (2008) *In the Realm of Hungry Ghosts: Close Encounters and Addiction*. Berkeley, CA: North Atlantic Books.

Shea, P. (2015) *Alchemy of the Extraordinary: A Journey into the Heart of the Meridian Matrix*. Asheville, NC: Peter Shea, Soul Pivot Press.

Van Der Kolk, B. (2014) *The Body Keeps the Score: Mind, Brain and Body in the Transformation of Trauma*. London: Penguin Books.

Index

Sub-headings in *italics* indicate tables.

acupuncture points
  acupuncture points to support
    the Hun 50–1
  acupuncture points to support
    the Po 47–8
  acupuncture points to support
    the Shen 57–8
  acupuncture points to support
    the Yi 53–4
  acupuncture points to support
    the Zhi 55–6
addiction 40–1
Ah Shi points 201
Alexander Technique 95
allostatic load 23
anxiety 24, 25–6, 45, 95,
  129–30, 136, 144
archetypes 58–60
  elemental archetypes of the
    Divergent channels 183–7
armoring 46, 71, 74–5
arthritis 40
assimilation 115
attention 52, 108–9
auto-immune disorders 26, 175, 176

babies 79, 121–2, 214
beliefs 16, 31–2
  emotions 173
birth trauma 25, 78–9
Black Lives Matter 210

blood and qi 24, 39, 48, 52, 105,
  108–9, 114–15, 118, 216
body awareness 94, 95
body memory 46, 79, 81, 82, 187
body-mind 32
boundaries 66, 113, 148
brain function 21–8
  triune brain 28–30
  Wei, Ying and Yuan qi 30–2
breathing 43–7, 95, 140, 202
  belly breathing 44–5
  exhale longer than the inhale 45
Buddhism 16
bullying 23–4

cancer 33–4, 133, 167
candidiasis 154
cardiovascular exercise 140
catecholamine 27
challenges 15–18, 236
change 21, 37–8, 149–50
channel system of acupuncture 34–5
  less is more 65–6
childbirth 27–8
children 44, 70–1, 123, 214–15
  childhood trauma 124
Chinese Medicine 24–5, 61, 94,
  238–9
Chödrön, Pema 16, 17
Chong mai 136, 212, 216,
  217, 220, 232–3

chronic conditions 22–3, 26, 34
   chronic fatigue 135–6
   development 38–41
   Divergent channels 172
   sinews 72
collective unconscious 49
compassion 66, 113, 128
consciousness 15, 56–7, 109, 236, 239
Corporeal Soul *see* Po
Cosmos 56, 58, 238
Covid-19 pandemic 60,
      77–8, 112, 207–10
criticism 131–2
Curious Organs 215–16

Dai mai 18, 39, 87, 213, 223, 234, 237–8
   consolidating 218–19
   Dai mai case study 226–32
   draining 219
   latency 217–18
danger 21–3
degenerative diseases 22, 26, 34,
      39, 175, 206, 232, 237
dependency 121–2
depression 24, 26, 135, 144
deprivation 121–2, 125, 126–7
Destiny 167
determination 54
diet 40, 105–6, 147–8
   self-help 156
digestion 52–3, 105–7, 147–8, 236–7
   aiding digestion 152–3
Divergent channels 18, 39,
      163–4, 237, 238
   assessing the zones 200–1
   conditions 175–6, 189–90, 191–2,
         192–3, 194, 195–6, 197, 205–6
   confluences 188–98
   Divergent channel case study 203–5
   elemental archetypes of the
         Divergent channels 183–7
   Gall Bladder and Liver
         confluence 190–2
   keys to self-help 202–3
   Large Intestine and Lung
         confluence 196–7
   mood vs temperament 167–74
   nature of Wei qi and Yuan qi 164–7
   Opening points of confluences 199–200

San Jiao and Pericardium
      confluence 195–6
Small Intestine and Heart
      confluence 193–4
Stomach and Spleen confluence 192–3
treating the Divergent
      channels 198–201
upper and lower meeting points
      174–6
*Upper and lower meeting points
      of confluences* 199
upper and lower meeting points of
      the six confluences 199–200
Urinary Bladder and Kidney
      confluence 188–90
why choose a Divergent
      treatment? 205–6
zonal theory 177–83
dreams 48–9
Du mai 86, 120, 212, 216, 221, 232–3
   Du mai Luo (Du-1) 137–8
   DU-4/Ming Men 56

Earth 59
East Asian Medicine 24–5, 61, 94
eating disorders 24
Eight Extraordinary Vessels (8 EV) 18,
      120, 133, 136, 137, 207–19, 238
   Chong mai 220
   Dai mai 223
   Dai mai case study 226–32
   Du mai 221
   Essential oils for use with the 8 EV 226
   keys to self-help 225–6
   Ren mai 220
   treatments 223–5
   why choose an 8 EV treatment? 232–4
   Yang Qiao 213, 222–3
   Yang Wei 221–2
   Yin Qiao 213, 222
   Yin Wei 221
elements 183–7, 238
   Earth 52, 60, 148, 150, 185
   Fire 59–60, 185–6
   Metal 46, 60, 186
   Water 54, 60, 183–4
   Wood 49, 58, 60, 184–5
emotions 23–4, 31, 56–7, 60, 167–8
   beliefs 173

Divergent channel confluences 190,
192, 193, 194, 196, 197
feel your feelings 140
Sinew channel treatments 92–4
Wei qi 168
Ying qi 107–8, 167–8
Yuan qi 168
empathy 66, 113, 128
Epsom salt soaks 96
essential oils 225
Essential oils for use with the 8 EV 226
Ethereal Soul see Hun
experiences 114–17, 120–1
context 115
overwhelming experiences 136–7

failure 153–4
Farrell, Y. 219
Feldenkrais 95
fibromyalgia 133–4
fitting in 111–13
five spirits 43, 58–60, 157
Hun/Ethereal Soul 48–51
Po/Corporeal Soul 43–8
Shen 56–8
Yi/thought 51–4
Zhi 54–6
Fruehauf, Heiner 154
Fu (yang) organs 31, 107, 116

Gall Bladder 25, 84
Gall Bladder Divergent channel
178–9, 190–2
Gall Bladder Luo (GB-37) 133–4
GB-25/Jing Men 56
gratitude 16–17, 18
grounding 148–50
growth 32, 39, 40–1
spiritual growth 50
Gu qi 52
Gu syndrome 154–6, 222
five Gu treatment 155–6
Gu syndrome case study 158–60

hangovers 116
he-sea points 91
Heart 18, 56, 60, 82, 84, 108–10,
113, 115, 166, 213
Heart Divergent channel 180, 193–4
Heart Luo (Ht-5) 127–8

Heavens 56, 238, 239
Herman, Aimée 43
human brain see neo-cortex
Hun 48–50, 54, 55, 58, 60, 79
acupuncture points to support
the Hun 50–1
Hun She/Abode of the Hun 51
hypervigilance 33, 44–5

I Ching 157
ideation 51–2
immune system 23, 26, 30–1, 175, 176
independence 127, 130–1
input 106–7
reducing 73–4, 95
intention 52, 54
interdependence 131
intergenerational trauma 25–6

jing 46, 106, 136–7, 166, 210,
211, 214, 215, 217
jing-river points 91
jing-well points 90, 201
jiu (number nine) 61–2
Jue Yin 87, 89
assessing 200
Liver and Pericardium Divergent
channels 181
right to occupy 182–3
Jung, Carl 15

Kidney(s) 54, 55, 84, 92, 106, 166
Kidney Divergent channel
180, 188–90
Kidney Luo (Ki-4) 114, 130–1
Ki-16/Huang Shu 48
Ki-22/Bu Lang 55
Ki-23/Shen Feng 53
Ki-24/Ling Xu 51
Ki-25/Shen Cang 57
Ki-26/Yu Zhong 47

labor 27–8
Large Intestine 84
Large Intestine Divergent
channel 179–80, 196–7
Large Intestine Luo (LI-6) 123–4
latency 18–19, 32, 34, 147
auto-immune disorders 176

latency *cont.*
  Dai mai 217–18
  Divergent channels 170–4, 198
  Eight Extraordinary Vessels
      (8 EV) 211–12
  latency creation 38–40, 60
  Luo-collateral system 114–22
  releasing latency 62–3
Laughing Qi Gong 140
leaky gut 107, 155
LGBTQ community 112–13
Li Dong Yuan 147
lifestyle 24–5, 40, 94, 108, 147–8
Liver 48–50, 81, 84, 92, 96, 116
  acupuncture points to support
      the Hun 50–1
  Liver Divergent channel 181, 190–2
  Liver Luo (Lv-5) 134–5
  Lv-13/Zhang Men 53–4
  Lv-14/Qi Men 51
loneliness 46
Los Angeles, USA 75–7
Lothian, J.A. 27
Lu, H.C. 163
Lung(s) 43, 54, 78, 84, 92, 96
  acupuncture points to support
      the Po 47–8
  Lung Divergent channel 180, 196–7
  Lung Luo (Lu-7) 122–3, 133
  Lu-1/Zhong Fu 47
  Lu-2/Yung Men 47
  Lu-3/Tian Fu 48
Luo-collateral system 18, 39, 113,
      114–22, 147, 237, 238
  conditions 118–19, 144
  Deep Luos 117
  Du mai Luo (Du-1) 137–8
  flows 120–1
  Gall Bladder Luo (GB-37) 133–4
  Heart Luo (Ht-5) 127–8
  keys to self-help 140
  Kidney Luo (Ki-4) 130–1
  Large Intestine Luo (LI-6) 123–4
  Liver Luo (Lv-5) 134–5
  Longitudinal Luos 117–18, 110, 138
  Lung Luo (Lu-7) 122–3, 133
  Luo-collateral case study 140–4
  Luo vessels 114–17, 119–22,
      138–9, 144–5
  pathology symptoms 118–19

  Pericardium Luo (Pc-6) 131–2
  Ren mai Luo (Ren-15) 137
  San Jiao Luo (Sj-5) 132–3
  Small Intestine Luo (SI-7) 128–9
  Spleen Luo (Sp-4) 125–7
  Spleen Luo (Sp-21) 135–6
  Stomach Luo (St-40) 124–5
  Stomach Luo (Xu Li) 136–7
  Transverse Luos 117
    treating the Luos 138–9
  Urinary Bladder Luo (UB-58)
      129–30
  why choose a Luo treatment? 144–5
Lyme disease 154

Maclean, Paul D. 28–9
Magic Square 61
Maitrī 16
mammalian brain 29, 30, 55
Mayan Oracle 157
midline points 201
mind *see* Shen
mindfulness 202
Ming Men 54
Miraculous Pivot 61
mood 167–74
Moreland, E. 154

natural world 74, 96
neo-cortex 29–30, 57
nine recommendations to
      practitioners 62–7
Nourishing Earth School (Spleen
      and Stomach School) 147–8
nutrition 24

Observer 57, 65
Observer: engaging the
      Observer 203, 226
orderliness 128–9
Other 163

pain 33–4, 62, 237, 239–40
  body memory 82
  Divergent channels 172––3
  patient's perception 63–4, 135–6
past-life experiences 49

Pericardium 18, 84, 87, 108, 109–10,
    115, 120, 130–2, 135, 137, 213, 237
  Pericardium Divergent
      channel 181, 195–6
  Pericardium Luo (Pc-6) 131–2
personality types 24–5
Pilates 95
Po 43–7, 54, 55, 60, 78, 123, 164
  acupuncture points to support
      the Po 47–8
  that which is most valuable is
      least substantial 47
  Wei qi and Po 78–80
post-traumatic stress disorder (PTSD) 26
practitioners and patients 62–7
predictability 38
Primary channels 18, 102, 116,
    119, 147–54, 237, 238
  conditions 160–1
  Gu syndrome 154–6
  Gu syndrome case study 158–60
  keys to self-help 156–8
  why choose a Primary channel
      treatment? 160–1

qi and blood 24, 39, 48, 52, 105,
    108–9, 114–15, 118, 216
quality of life 22–3, 34
Quinn, B. 154

redundancy 238
referrals 64–5
relationships 31, 110–11, 237
  therapeutic relationship 62–7
Ren mai 120, 212, 216, 220, 232–3
  Ren mai Luo (Ren-15) 137
  Ren-12/Zhong Wan 54
  Ren-14/Ju Que 57
  Ren-15/Jiu Wei 58
reproductive decisions 112
reptilian brain 29, 30, 37, 45, 153, 177
resistance 37–41, 64
  practitioners' resistance 66–7
resources 15, 18, 22–4, 32, 33,
    55, 106, 210–11, 238–9
  latency 34, 39–41

safety 27–8, 38
San Jiao 132–3, 151, 166

San Jiao Divergent channel
    178–9, 195–6
San Jiao Luo (Sj-5) 132–3
sciatica 85
Self 15, 31, 41, 59, 60, 65, 71, 80,
    133, 135, 137, 163, 164, 221
  sense of Self 166–7, 217
  temperament 169
self-acceptance 16–17, 235–6
self-awareness 56, 113, 127, 128
self-preservation 15, 18–19, 34, 239
  resistance 37–41
  sinews 69–78
Shao Yang 86, 88, 133, 221
  assessing 200
  Gall Bladder and San Jiao
      Divergent channels 178–9
  right to decide 182, 183
Shao Yin 86, 89, 127
  assessing 200
  Heart and Kidney Divergent
      channels 180
  right to measure/impart value 182,
      183
Shen 29, 43, 48, 56–7, 59–60,
    79, 109, 166
  acupuncture points to support
      the Shen 57–8
shock 24, 188, 205
shu-stream points 91
Sinew channels 17–18, 39, 176
  assessing the sinews 88–90
  conditions 102
  creating a Sinew channel
      treatment 90–4
  emotional trauma 82
  external factors 80, 82
  keys to self-help 94–6
  meeting points 85, 90
  organ imbalances 83–4
  organ pathology 81
  overuse or improper use 81, 82–3
  physical trauma 80–1
  Sinew channel meeting points 85
  Sinew channel treatment
      case study 96–101
  Sinew groupings 84
  sinews and self-preservation 69–78
  Six Cutaneous Zones 85–7, 177
  Wei qi and Po 78–80

Sinew channels *cont.*
  why choose a Sinew channel
      treatment? 102–3
  yang sinews 87
  yin sinews 88
Six Cutaneous Zones 85–7, 177
  constitutional rights 181–3
  Jue Yin 181
  Shao Yang 178–9
  Shao Yin 180
  Tai Yang 177–8
  Tai Yin 180
  Yang Ming 179–80
sleep 48–9, 56, 165–6
Small Intestine 84, 85
  Small Intestine Divergent
      channel 177–8, 193–4
  Small Intestine Luo (SI-7) 128–9
small intestine bacterial
      overgrowth (SIBO) 107
Spleen 51, 52, 55, 84, 108–9,
      113, 115, 116, 120
  Spleen Divergent channel 180, 192–3
  Spleen Luo (Sp-4) 125–7
  Spleen Luo (Sp-21) 135–6
stillness 202
Stomach 52, 84, 92, 120
  Stomach Divergent channel
      179–80, 192–3
  Stomach Luo (St-40) 124–5
  Stomach Luo (Xu Li) 136–7
  St-36/Zu San Li 54
stress 16, 23–8, 210
  hypervigilance 33
survival 17–19, 163–4, 237
  brain function 21–8
  cost of survival 32–5, 38–41
  redundancy 238

Tai Yang 85–6, 88, 127, 165
  assessing 200
  right to act 181, 183
  Urinary Bladder and Small Intestine
      Divergent channels 177–8
Tai Yin 89
  assessing 200
  Lung and Spleen Divergent
      channels 180
  right to embrace/accept 182, 183

Tarot 157
temperament 15
  mood vs temperament 167–74
therapeutic relationship 62–7
thought *see* Yi
threats 37–8, 73, 129–30
  bracing against threats 70–1, 236–7
thriving 15–16, 27, 34–5
trauma 18–19, 23–5, 46, 60, 124, 214–15
  body memory 187
  letting go of trauma 65
  Sinew channels 80–1, 82
Triple Burner 195
Triple Warmer 84, 131
triune brain 28–30

Universe 59, 238
Urinary Bladder 84, 85, 87
  Urinary Bladder Divergent
      channel 177–8, 188–90
  Urinary Bladder Luo (UB-58) 129–30
  UB-42/Po Hu 47
  UB-44/Shen Tang 57
  UB-47/Hun Men 50
  UB-49/Yi She 53
  UB-52/Zhi Shi 55

Wei Mai 212
Wei qi (defensive qi) 29, 30–1, 37,
      41, 153, 161, 163–4, 236, 238
  creating a Sinew channel
      treatment 90–4
  hypervigilance 44–5
  keys to self-help 94–6, 202
  nature of Wei qi and Yuan qi 164–7
  sinews 69–70, 72–5, 77–8, 89–90
  Wei qi and Po 78–80
  Ying qi 106, 107, 108, 115–16, 171

xi-cleft points 91, 201

Yang Ming 86, 88
  assessing 200
  right to demand/need 182, 183
  Stomach and Large Intestine
      Divergent channels 179–80
Yang Qiao 213, 222–3, 234
yang sinews 87

Yang Wei 212–13, 221–2, 233–4
Yi 37, 51–3, 54, 55, 59, 60,
    108, 115, 149. 216
  acupuncture points to support
      the Yi 53–4
Yin Qiao 213, 222, 234
yin sinews 88
Yin Wei 136, 213, 221, 233
Ying qi (nutritive qi) 29, 30,
    31, 37, 41, 48, 52, 115–16,
    165, 216, 232–3, 236
  digestion, emotion and
      interaction 105–14
  keys to self-help 140, 156–8
  Luo-collateral system 114–17,
    120–1, 125, 134–5

Primary channels 147, 160
  treating the Luos 138, 144
yoga 95
Yuan level points 201
Yuan qi (source qi) 29, 30, 31–2, 41, 57,
    65, 113, 132–3, 161, 163–4, 236
  Eight Extraordinary Vessels (8 EV) 210
  keys to self-help 202–3
  nature of Wei qi and Yuan qi 164–7
Yuan Shen 210
Yuen, Jeffrey 47, 155, 225–6

Zhi 29, 54–5, 60, 166
  acupuncture points to support
      the Zhi 55–6